Introduction to the Professional Aspects of Medical Physics

Kenneth R. Hogstrom, PhD
Professor of Radiation Physics

and

John L. Horton, PhD
Associate Professor of Radiation Physics

Department of Radiation Physics
Division of Radiation Oncology
The University of Texas M. D. Anderson Cancer Center
Houston, TX

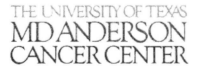

THE UNIVERSITY OF TEXAS
MD ANDERSON
CANCER CENTER

The University of Texas M. D. Anderson Cancer Center
Houston, TX

Library of Congress Cataloguing in Publication Data:

Library of Congress Catalog Card Number: 99-63579
ISBN: 0-944838-89-8

Printed in the United States of America

Dedication

This lecture series and book are dedicated to the future of medical physics—today's students, residents, and trainees.

Preface

Most recent graduates of medical physics training programs are highly focused on the scientific and technical aspects of medical physics as they begin their first job as a professional medical physicist. To the surprise of many, they are suddenly cast in the midst of a highly complicated political and administrative environment. Many are suddenly exposed to fiscal issues, administrative problems, conflict resolution, and a variety of other professional issues. They then have to learn the other side of medical physics. Also, trainees about to graduate begin looking for the position for which they have spent long, hard hours training, but have few clues as to how to proceed or what to look for. The realization of these issues by a few of our more recent students and graduates led them to request some training in this area. Hence was the genesis of this lecture series and book. This book is intended to be used as the text for a 1-semester-hour course for graduate students or as supplementary reading for resident trainees. However, practicing medical physicists might also find it informative and useful as it provides reminders about professional information and behavior.

It was decided that a documented lecture series by some of the top professionals in our field would be the quickest and most effective way to introduce trainees to the professional aspects of medical physics. We put together a detailed program of 15 lectures that we felt would provide a comprehensive introduction. For most lecture topics, we could identify multiple qualified speakers, but we focused on speakers who were active in the specific area through our professional societies and often professionals who had worked or trained at The University of Texas M. D. Anderson Cancer Center, Houston, TX. These lectures were presented in 1997 to medical physics students and faculty of The University of Texas Health Science Center at Houston Graduate School of Biomedical Sciences through the Medical Physics Seminars of M. D. Anderson Cancer Center's Department of Radiation Physics.

The material presented in the lectures and these proceedings introduce contemporary views on a number of topics important to the profession of medical physics. In time, conditions will change, and this material will need to be updated. At that time, we hope that either M. D. Anderson Cancer Center or another major training center will be in a position to repeat this process.

The book can be divided into six major sections: professional organizations, professional credentials, job opportunities, professional job skills, financial issues, and technical references. The first section provides information on the three organizations that support the professional needs of medical physicists and to which most professionals are members: the American Association of Physicists in Medicine, the American College of Medical Physics, and the American College of Radiology. The second section addresses the credentials of professional medical physicists: certification by the American Board of Radiology and by the American Board of Medical Physics, state licensure, and hospital credentialing. The third section speaks on job opportunities by explaining staffing in radiology and radiation oncology departments and by offering wisdom on how to search for a job. The fourth section provides insight on how to interact successfully in the work environment, first recommending a behavior that will allow one to advance in their first job and then addressing how to interact with administrators, physicians, and other allied health professionals. The health care marketplace is strongly driven by financial aspects, and the fifth section discusses billing for physics procedures and managed care. Individual as well as institutional financial protection is important, so the topic of professional liability is covered. In the sixth and final section, we return to the technical side of medical physics and offer a discussion of the vast amount of technical information presently available, how to access it, and how it should be used.

We hope that this introduction to the professional aspects of medical physics will smooth the transition from the training environment to the professional environment and allow the medical physicist to be more successful and of more value to his or her respective institution. Lastly, we hope that these topics will help teach the young medical physicist that early support and activity in their professional societies will benefit their profession and ultimately themselves. The profession of medical physics was not handed to us but rather has matured as a result of the selfless participation of many medical physicists like you!

This lecture series and book would not have been possible without the contributions of so many. First, we are indebted for the financial support of the American College of Medical Physics, the American Association of Physicists in Medicine, and M. D. Anderson Cancer Center. Support from M. D. Anderson was made possible by the 1995 Faculty Achievement Award in Education given to Kenneth Hogstrom. Second, we are particularly grateful to the speakers for the selfless giving of their time and effort in travelling to Houston, TX to deliver their lectures and in writing manuscripts. Third, we cannot thank enough Vickie Williams, scientific editor in the Department of Scientific Publications at M. D. Anderson for her incredible talent in editing the manuscripts into a cohesive and eloquent presentation. Fourth, we are especially grateful to Georgeanne Moore, educational coordinator in the Department of Radiation Physics at M. D. Anderson, for her administrative skill in coordinating speaker visits, for her word processing skill as the book was edited and structured prior to printing, and for her management skills in tying up a number of loose ends. Lastly, we want to acknowledge our graduate students for their active support of the lectures, for meeting with the individual lecturers, and for their youthful vigor and inquisitiveness that stimulated us all.

Kenneth R. Hogstrom, PhD
John L. Horton, PhD

About the Editors

Kenneth R. Hogstrom, PhD

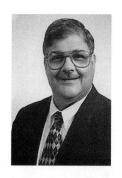

Kenneth R. Hogstrom completed the requirements for the PhD in Physics from Rice University in Houston, TX in 1976. From 1973 to 1974, between his MS in Physics from the University of Houston and his PhD studies, Dr. Hogstrom worked at The University of Texas M. D. Anderson Hospital and Tumor Institute (now The University of Texas M. D. Anderson Cancer Center) in Houston as a Research Assistant on the neutron therapy project. From 1976 to 1979, Dr. Hogstrom worked as a Senior Research Assistant for the University of New Mexico Cancer Research and Treatment Center, participating in the pion therapy project at the Los Alamos National Laboratory. In 1979, he rejoined M. D. Anderson Cancer Center as an Assistant Professor in the Department of Physics. In 1986, he was appointed Chairman of the newly formed Department of Radiation Physics in the Division of Radiation Oncology, and in 1987, he was promoted to Professor of Radiation Physics. Dr. Hogstrom is an established researcher, having published over 100 journal articles and book chapters. His contributions in electron-beam dose algorithms and treatment techniques have resulted in numerous honors and awards, including the P. H. and Fay Etta Robinson Professorship in Cancer Research. Since 1985, Dr. Hogstrom has served as Director of the Medical Physics Program at The University of Texas Health Science Center at Houston Graduate School of Biomedical Sciences, where he also is an instructor and mentor. His interest in and contributions to education resulted in his receiving the 1995 Faculty Achievement Award in Education at M. D. Anderson. Dr. Hogstrom has made numerous professional contributions, having served on many committees and task groups of the American Association of Physicists in Medicine (AAPM) and the American College of Medical Physics (ACMP) and on the Commission on Accreditation of Medical Physics Education Programs, Inc. He is a Fellow of the AAPM and ACMP and is the 1999 President elect of the AAPM.

John L. Horton, PhD

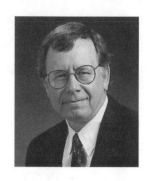

John L. Horton received his PhD in Physics from The University of Texas in Austin, TX, in 1971. Subsequently, he was an Atomic Energy Control Board postdoctoral fellow at the University of Manitoba cyclotron laboratory and a National Academy of Sciences Resident Research Associate at the tandem Van de Graaff facility of the U.S. Army Ballistics Research Laboratory. Dr. Horton received training in medical physics as a postdoctoral fellow in the Department of Physics at The University of Texas M. D. Anderson Hospital and Tumor Institute (now The University of Texas M. D. Anderson Cancer Center) in Houston, TX from 1975 to 1976. He spent 1 year at M. D. Anderson Hospital as an Assistant in Physics before becoming Chief Radiation Physicist at the Cleveland Clinic in 1977. In 1985, he rejoined M. D. Anderson as Chief of the Section of Clinical Dosimetry in the Department of Radiation Physics. Dr. Horton is presently Associate Professor, Leader of the Brachytherapy Services Group, and Deputy Chair of the Department of Radiation Physics. Dr. Horton is best known for his clinical expertise as a therapeutic radiological physicist. He has served as an oral examiner in radiation therapy physics for both the American Board of Medical Physics and the American Board of Radiology. He is also an established academician. Dr. Horton has published one textbook on radiation therapy physics, was co-organizer of an American College of Medical Physics (ACMP)-sponsored conference on quality assurance in radiation therapy physics and co-editor of the conference proceedings, has written several chapters in radiation therapy physics texts, and has published numerous scientific journal articles. He is also an active instructor and mentor in the Medical Physics Program of The University of Texas Health Science Center at Houston Graduate School of Biomedical Sciences. Dr. Horton's significant professional contributions include having served on the American Association of Physicists in Medicine (AAPM) Radiation Therapy Committee, the ACMP Board of Chancellors, and as ACMP newsletter editor. He is a Fellow of the AAPM and ACMP. He is currently a member of the Human Resources Committee of the American Society for Therapeutic Radiology and Oncology and Associate Editor of Radiation Oncology Physics for the *Journal of Applied Clinical Medical Physics*.

Table of Contents

Professional Organizations

American Association of Physicists in Medicine: A Summary of Roles and Activities[*]

Bhudatt R. Paliwal, PhD

Department of Human Oncology, University of Wisconsin, Madison, WI

Abstract. Four decades have elapsed since the American Association of Physicists in Medicine (AAPM) was formed in 1958. During this period, the association has matured and grown significantly. The educational, scientific, professional, and administrative committees of the AAPM and the organizations of the executive services have become extremely elaborate. This chapter provides a snapshot of some of these activities. It is intended to assist the new and younger professionals to rapidly become familiar with some of the important structures and processes of the AAPM.

1. History and mission

The application of physical sciences to the field of medicine is probably as old as the medical profession itself; indeed, the marriage of these fields was documented 5 centuries ago in the works of Leonardo de Vinci. Although over the past century significant interest in medical physics has emerged, the true identity of this profession did not come about until the middle of the 20th century. For decades, physicists involved in research, teaching, and the application of medical physics met informally at the annual meetings of the Radiological Society of North America (RSNA). Gail Adams, PhD, the first formal president of the newly formed American Association of Physicists in Medicine (AAPM), took office in 1958 and held the first AAPM meeting at the time of the RSNA annual meeting. There were approximately 150 AAPM members at that time. By the 1960s, the AAPM had grown to the point that it held a separate annual meeting in the summer while continuing to meet with the RSNA in the fall. Today, the AAPM has over 4200 members. This number continues to increase 3% to 5% each year. The AAPM maintains its headquarters in College Park, MD, and is a resident member society of the American Institute of Physics (AIP).

In the late 1950s, medical physics rapidly became a distinct academic science, and thus, the AAPM had to assume a broader role as a professional as well as scientific and educational organization. Accordingly, the articles-of-incorporation of the AAPM state that its purpose is to: promote the application of physics to medicine and biology, encourage interest and training in medical physics and related fields, and prepare and disseminate technical information in medical physics and related fields.

---

[*] Adapted from A Guide to the AAPM (AAPM 1996).

More recently, an Ad Hoc Strategic Planning Committee recommended the development of a mission statement for the AAPM that also would include the following purposes: to ensure that the professional interests of all members are represented and to promote, encourage, and facilitate high-quality medical physics services for patients.

2. Organizational structure

2.1. Board of directors

The board of directors governs the AAPM and is the policy-making body of the organization. The board is composed of 5 elected officers, 12 board members at-large (elected by the entire membership), and 20 regional chapter representatives (elected by members of each chapter). Ex-officio members of the board include the executive director and the 2 representatives to the AIP governing board. The 5 elected officers—president, president-elect, chairman of the board (past president), secretary, and treasurer—have specific and general functions that encompass the overall activities of the organization. The officers and the executive director make up the executive committee of the board (EXCOM), which meets during the AAPM and RSNA annual meetings and, typically, three more times throughout the year. One meeting usually takes place at AAPM headquarters and includes three council chairs and is devoted to long-range planning.

2.2. Councils and committees

Most activities of the AAPM are conducted through the voluntary work of councils and committees. All nonadministrative committees of the AAPM function under one of three councils: education, professional, and science. The routine business functions of the AAPM are handled by the administrative committees. The councils and committees meet at least twice a year, once at the AAPM annual meeting and again at either the annual RSNA meeting or at the annual American Society for Therapeutic Radiology and Oncology (ASTRO) meeting. Each year, the president-elect recommends, to the board of directors, annual appointment of committee and subcommittee chairpersons and members to each group. Chairpersons and members serve 3-year terms. Committee chairpersons in turn appoint task-group chairpersons and task-group members and advise the president elect on appointments to task-group and subcommittee positions. Members of all councils, committees, subcommittees, and task groups are listed in the annual membership directory. New committee reports are available on the AAPM World Wide Web site: www.aapm.org.

Volunteering for a committee or a task group is an effective way to become involved in the AAPM. Members may write to the president-elect, a committee chairperson, or a council chairperson to request an appointment.

2.2.1. Education council and committees. The education council and committees oversee, monitor, and facilitate programs offered by the AAPM to educate and train medical physicists. The council coordinates AAPM educational activities with those of other organizations, such as the RSNA, the American College of Medical Physics, the American College of Radiology, and ASTRO. Committees of the education council include:

- Continuing education: provides an opportunity for continuing education of members, including planning, preparing, and executing the annual summer-school program and other continuing-education programs

- Education and training of medical physicists: collects statistical information on trainees, provides training guidelines, and promotes programs dealing with the training of medical physicists

- Public education: promotes public education in matters concerning medical physics; formulates, collects, and distributes information about the practice of medical physics to the public

- Training of radiologists: collects and distributes information related to medical physics training of radiologists

- Training of technologists: promotes upgrading of physics teaching in technology training programs and provides liaison with other societies

2.2.2. Professional council and committees. The professional council and committees address professional concerns of the membership and the medical physics profession. Committees of the professional council include:

- Ethics: provides advice on matters relating to the ethical practice of medical physics; hears cases regarding ethical practice by individual medical physicists

- Legislation and regulation: provides advice on legislation and regulatory activities at the local, state, and federal levels; formulates and recommends the position of the AAPM to the board of directors

- Professional information and clinical relations: advises the AAPM on matters concerning the clinical practice of medical physics, informs the public and other professionals of the contributions of clinical medical physics, conducts surveys that address the clinical role of medical physicists, and supervises the annual AAPM salary survey

2.2.3. Science council and committees. The science council examines specific areas of medical physics to determine advancement mechanisms, addresses scientific questions, and collates and assesses data. Committees of the science council include:

- Biological effects: collects and distributes information concerning the biological effects of radiation, especially as used in diagnostic and therapeutic medical procedures

- Computer: provides advice on the use of computers in medical physics, promotes use of computers to facilitate communication among members, and acts as a resource to the headquarters staff for tasks regarding electronic mail and publishing

- Diagnostic x-ray imaging: provides advice on medical applications of x-ray imaging modalities such as radiography, fluoroscopy, computed tomography, and digital radiography

- General medical physics: provides advice on emerging non-ionizing, therapeutic, and diagnostic modalities

- Magnetic resonance: provides advice on medical application of nuclear magnetic resonance imaging techniques

- Nuclear medicine: provides advice on application of physics to nuclear medicine

- Radiation protection: provides advice on matters concerning radiation protection and responds to federal- and state-agency actions, regulations, or proposed regulations concerning radiation protection matters

- Radiation therapy: provides advice on application of physics in radiation therapy

- Research: provides advice on research activities of the AAPM membership and how to assist the membership in obtaining financial support for independent research

- Ultrasound: provides advice on application of ultrasound imaging techniques to medicine

2.2.4. Administrative committees. The administrative committees encompass all other organizational relationships, operational functions, and governing aspects of the AAPM. These committees include:

- Annual meeting coordination: coordinates and supervises the planning and execution of the annual meeting, develops and updates guidelines for the annual meeting, and evaluates sites for future meetings

- Awards and honors: recommends candidates for AAPM awards and honors to the board of directors

- Development: coordinates efforts to solicit donations to the AAPM education fund and other research education funds, develops and administers a planned giving endowment program, and recommends dispersal of education and research funds

- Executive: serves as the advisory cabinet to the president and the AAPM and carries out recommendations to the board of directors

- Finance: advises board of directors on all monetary affairs of the AAPM (chaired by the treasurer)

- History: advises board of directors concerning history of medical physics and the AAPM; proposes methods and policies to preserve history recorded in documents, photographs, personal papers, professional memorabilia, scientific records, and equipment

- International affairs: advises board of directors on activities of an international nature conducted by either individuals or committees on behalf of the AAPM

- Investment advisory: evaluates various investment opportunities available to the AAPM and advises the board of directors and executive committee concerning investments of AAPM financial resources

- Journal business management: advises board of directors on activities of the *Medical Physics* journal

- Membership: examines applications for new membership and changes in existing membership, determines the appropriate class of membership, and approves or rejects an application based on the information submitted

- Nominating: prepares a slate of potential candidates for AAPM officers and board members at-large for approval by the board of directors

- Program: organizes the annual meeting program by selecting speakers, symposia, scientific abstracts, scientific exhibits, and other aspects of the program; collaborates with the RSNA program committee

- Publications: reviews and recommends policy and financial matters regarding AAPM publications, including scientific, educational, technical, and administrative reports; official brochures; and all other printed or duplicated matter

- Regional organization: assists groups of members in establishing regional chapters and junior chapters

- Research: provides advice about the research activities of the AAPM membership and makes recommendations for educational activities that will help the membership to obtain financial support for independent research

- Rules: interprets and develops language for board-approved modifications to articles-of-incorporation, bylaws, and rules of the AAPM

- Special interest groups: provides association and communication mechanisms for groups that share common medical physics interests, such as computers

(computers and medical physics special interest group, CAMPSIG) and nuclear medicine (nuclear medicine special interest group, NUCSIG).

3. Sponsorship

The AAPM is a sponsor of the American Board of Radiology, which certifies medical physicists as well as their physician colleagues. Board certification is encouraged by the AAPM as a means of demonstrating entry-level competence and experience. The AAPM also sponsors the Commission on Accreditation of Medical Physics Education Programs, Inc. (CAMPEP), which accredits graduate and resident education programs in medical physics. The AAPM also encourages its members to maintain professional competency by taking advantage of continuing-education opportunities accredited by CAMPEP, such as annual meetings, summer schools, and sponsored symposia.

4. Membership

All memberships are renewed annually and follow the calendar-year schedule. AAPM membership status should reflect a current member's career position. Members are required to change membership status as their position in the medical physics profession changes. There are five categories of membership.

4.1. Full membership

Full membership is granted to scientists or engineers working in the field of medical physics who meet the training and experience requirements of the AAPM. One of the following educational requirements must be met:

- PhD or DSc degree in physical science plus 1 year minimum experience in medical physics

- MA or MS degree in physical science plus 2 years minimum experience in medical physics

Experience may be reduced by 1 year if the person's postgraduate degree is from an AAPM-accredited medical physics program. In special cases, individuals who fail to meet these academic requirements but can demonstrate adequate experience and have contributed significantly to medical physics may be considered eligible for full membership.

4.2. Associate membership

Associate membership is granted to individuals working in areas of physics where there is no direct application to medicine or biology or individuals engaged in other than developmental aspects of equipment for biological or medical use.

4.3. Corresponding membership

Individuals residing overseas who meet the qualifications for full or associate membership may apply for corresponding membership

4.4. Junior membership

Applicants for junior membership must have a minimum of a BA or BS degree and be preparing to meet requirements for full membership.

4.5. Student membership

Membership may be granted to full-time students currently enrolled in full-time medical physics graduate programs.

5. Participation

The AAPM provides a variety of activities for members and non-members, including the following.

5.1. Meetings

The AAPM holds an annual meeting each summer. This 5-day meeting includes scientific sessions, technical displays, and abstract displays. In mid-November, the AAPM mails a call-for-papers requesting that abstracts be submitted by the first Friday in February for the upcoming summer's annual meeting. A call-for-works-in-progress is mailed a few months before the annual meeting. At the RSNA meeting each autumn, designated AAPM members are responsible for the Medical Physics Scientific Program, and as such, all AAPM individual members are invited to register for the RSNA meeting free of charge.

5.2. Summer school for professional enrichment

The AAPM hosts an annual summer-school program on a university campus in North America. The subject alternates each year between topics focusing on diagnostic and therapeutic applications for medical physics.

5.3. Committees

The AAPM's over 100 councils, committees, subcommittees, and task groups meet at least twice a year to discuss, determine, research, and publish information that is important to the profession of medical physics and to its practitioners. Over 50 task-group reports have been published by the AAPM. The reports are published in *Medical Physics* when appropriate, or they are published separately and mailed to all AAPM members. Each year, the AAPM president-elect calls for members to request committee assignments for the following year. The standard duration for a committee appointment is one 3-year term.

5.4. Affiliation with an AAPM regional chapter

There are 20 AAPM regional chapters. Each chapter holds its own meetings, elects its own officers, and sends a representative to the board of directors' meetings. To join a regional chapter, an individual must be a member of the AAPM.

5.5. Affiliation with the AIP and the International Organization of Medical Physics

The AAPM is a member society of the AIP and the International Organization of Medical Physics (IOMP), and as such, AAPM members receive free, with their paid membership, the AIP journal *Physics Today,* discounted subscriptions to *Physics in Medicine and Biology* and other AIP publications, and the semi-annual IOMP bulletin entitled *Medical Physics World.*

6. Benefits

The AAPM is an exceptionally rich resource for scientific and professional information, with something to offer individuals at all levels of membership. In addition to its milieu of knowledge and experience, the benefits of AAPM membership include:

- Monthly issues of *Medical Physics*, the AAPM journal
- Monthly issues of the AAPM placement bulletin
- Monthly issues of *Physics Today*, the AIP journal
- Reduced rates on all other AIP subscriptions
- Bi-monthly issues of the *AAPM Newsletter*
- 10 monthly mailings
- Reduced registration fees to the AAPM annual meeting
- Free registration to the RSNA meeting
- An annual membership directory
- An annual salary survey
- Participation on committees and task groups
- Free copies of task-group reports as published
- 20 regional chapters
- Emeritus membership
- Access to professional liability insurance

7. Communications

The AAPM communicates with its membership and other professional, scientific, and corporate organizations in a variety of ways.

7.1. Internet

The AAPM's Internet Web site address is www.aapm.org. This Web site contains large amounts of information about the activities of the AAPM. There are plans to provide considerably more scientific, educational, and professional material through this Web site in the future.

7.2. AAPM Newsletter

The *AAPM Newsletter* is distributed bi-monthly. The deadline for receipt of material for publication consideration is 6 weeks before the mailing date. The Editor, Robert Dixon, welcomes entries. You may contact him by phone at (910) 721-9171, by fax at (910) 721-0833, or by e-mail at brdcst@aol.com. He encourages authors to include a photograph. The newsletter is provided to all members free of additional charges.

7.3. Membership directory listing

The annual AAPM membership directory contains the current information for each calendar year: names of executive officers; dates of upcoming meetings; lists of the board of directors and regional chapter officers; the membership of councils, committees, and task groups; and the current version of the AAPM bylaws and rules. Each autumn, members are asked to provide a "directory address" for the alphabetical listing in the directory.

7.4. Professional information survey report

Each spring, the AAPM requests salary, benefits, and occupation data from each of its North American members. These data are analyzed and printed for disbursement to all AAPM members each June.

7.5. Placement bulletin

The AAPM Placement Bulletin or "Blue Sheets" is a monthly publication compiled by a member of the AAPM. Corporations and institutions who are seeking to hire a medical physicist or related professional (e.g., medical dosimetrist, accelerator engineer, postdoctoral fellow, or clinical resident) may place advertisements in the bulletin each month. Any AAPM member who is seeking employment may include a notice about himself or herself once every 6 months.

8. Financial basis

Financial support for AAPM activities is derived primarily from membership dues, annual meeting profits, educational program profits, publications, and interest on reserves. The membership donates substantial volunteer activity. More than 300 members serve on the science, professional, education, and administrative committees of the AAPM or act as liaisons between the AAPM and other scientific and government groups. In addition, the AAPM has 20 regional chapters that meet regularly to provide scientific and professional information to members.

9. Awards and fellowships

The AAPM has an extensive program through which the contributions of its members are recognized. Each year, the Awards and Honors Committee of the AAPM bestows its most distinguished award, the Coolidge Award, named after William D. Coolidge who in 1913 produced the first practical x-ray tube, which utilized a hot cathode. The Coolidge Award is the highest honor of the AAPM. It is given each year to an individual who has established a distinguished career in medical physics and has exerted a significant impact on the practice of medical physics. Other awards given annually by the AAPM are the Young Investigators Award, the AAPM/IPSM Travel Award, the AAPM Medical Physics Travel Award, the Farrington Daniels Award, the Sylvia Sorkin-Greenfield Award, and Achievement Awards. Also each year, the AAPM recognizes members as fellows for distinguished services to the organization.

The AAPM also has an active development program that provides funds to support the education and training of medical physicists. The AAPM awards fellowships that support stipends, tuition, and travel for students and residents enrolled in CAMPEP-accredited programs.

References

American Association of Physicists in Medicine (1996) A Guide to the AAPM. College Park, MD:AAPM

— (1998) American Association of Physicists in Medicine Directory. College Park, MD:AAPM

— (1998) History of the American Association of Physicists in Medicine 1958-1998. *Medical Physics* **25**

Bhudatt R. Paliwal, PhD

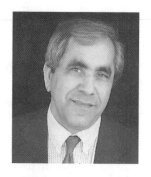

Bhudatt R. Paliwal received his PhD in Biophysics from The University of Texas Graduate School of Biomedical Sciences in Houston, TX in 1973. Upon graduation, Dr. Paliwal joined the Department of Radiology at the University of Wisconsin Center for Health Sciences in Madison, WI where he is now Professor in the Departments of Medical Physics and Human Oncology and Director of Radiation Therapy Physics in the Section of Radiation Oncology of the Department of Human Oncology. Dr. Paliwal served as Assistant and Associate Director for the Midwest Center for Radiologic Physics from 1974 to1980. Dr. Paliwal is an active researcher and has published over 100 papers in refereed journals. Dr. Paliwal is a Fellow of the AAPM and the International Atomic Energy Agency. He has served on and chaired many professional task groups and scientific review committees. He was President of the AAPM in 1996 and has served as Chair of the Board of Directors for the Commission on Accreditation of the Medical Physics Educational Programs, Inc. (CAMPEP).

The American College of Medical Physics: Why and How

Walter H. Grant III, PhD

Department of Radiology, Baylor College of Medicine, Houston, TX

Abstract. The American College of Medical Physics (ACMP) was formed in 1983 by medical physicists to address professional issues of concern to medical physicists. The organization was established with financial support from the American Association of Physicists in Medicine. The ACMP is governed by elected officers and members of the Board of Chancellors. Its councils and committees have contributed significantly to the profession of medical physics. The ACMP was the first organization (1986) to define the term "qualified medical physicist," which provided regulatory agencies with the terminology needed to identify the responsibilities of a physicist in their documentation. The ACMP has supported the certification of medical physicists by establishing the American Board of Medical Physics, a body composed solely of physicists to address the needs of physicists. The ACMP has supported licensure for medical physicists in Texas, Florida, California, and New York. To have a long and successful career, medical physicists must develop more than technical skills, and the ACMP offers them the opportunity to do so.

1. Introduction

I appreciate the opportunity to describe the American College of Medical Physics (ACMP) to young medical physicists. As the title explains, I have two messages for you. The first is that the medical physicist must be concerned with all aspects of his or her career, not just technical expertise. The other message is that the ACMP is the best vehicle to use to broaden one's knowledge about this field. I learned these lessons firsthand when I left the security of a large, academic physics group to work for a group of private practice physicians only to have the physicians disband abruptly. I needed skills to survive, skills other than the ability to calibrate machines and calculate doses. I was fortunate that the ACMP was coming into existence at this crucial time in my career. So, before I explain how the ACMP has already helped you and can continue to do so, let me review why I believe physicists need to expand their skill set to include expertise other than technical know-how.

2. Why you need other skills

Figure 1 was presented by Richard Grote, an author and management consultant, at the 13th ACMP Annual Meeting. Grote pointed out that laymen assume that experienced technical people have the skills required to perform their jobs, which is what the terms "certified" and "licensed" imply. As an example, he asked, "Why do you think your dry cleaner is the best?" It is not likely your answer will be based on the technical expertise of the workers. Your answer might be based on cost, convenience, personal interaction, or some other parameter, but probably not technical expertise (Grote 1996). As a medical physicist, your employer will expect you to manage people, write specifications for equipment purchases, train others, and, eventually, give guidance for future plans. Where will you get this training? You will get it from an organization that concerns itself with these types of subjects— the ACMP.

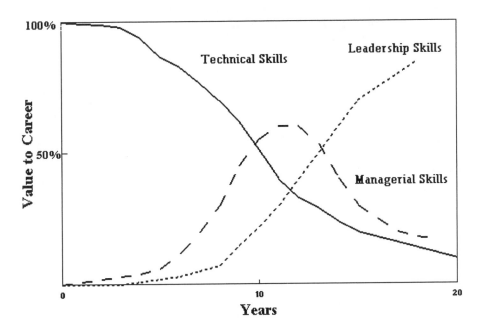

Figure 1.   The importance of different types of skills during a medical physicist's professional career. Reprinted with permission from Richard Grote.

3. Formation of the ACMP

The idea for a separate professional organization to address issues of importance to medical physicists began to be discussed by members of the American Association of Physicists in Medicine (AAPM) in 1972. The idea was affirmed by 69% of the membership. A committee was formed to make recommendations for the formalities of such an organization; they proposed the formation of the American Academy of Medical Physics. Instead, the AAPM created the Professional Council.

In 1979, another survey was taken of the AAPM membership to determine if the organization should be more active in attempting to influence legislation and regulation. The results were 311 for and 11 against. In 1981, the AAPM Ad Hoc Committee on Professionalism recommended the formation of the ACMP, and in November of that same year, the AAPM Board of Directors voted to provide $5000 to support the ACMP Constituting Board. In 1982, the AAPM Board of Directors voted to support the formation of the ACMP; the results were 26 for, 1 against, and 3 abstain.

In 1983, the ACMP Board of Chancellors was formed with at least one member from each AAPM chapter. This model for complementary professional and scientific societies was based on that of other radiological medical organizations, such as the American College of Radiology (ACR)/Radiological Society of North America (RSNA), in which the ACR serves as the professional arm and the RSNA as the scientific arm for diagnostic radiologists. Likewise, we have the ACR/American Society of Therapeutic Radiology and Oncology (ASTRO), in which ASTRO serves as the scientific arm for radiation oncologists.

4. ACMP structure

The ACMP has approximately 400 members. It is an ACR council member and is headquartered at the ACR office in Reston, VA. It is governed by the Board of Chancellors, which consists of its elected officers (chairman, immediate past chairman, vice chairman, secretary, and treasurer) and elected chancellors from nine geographical regions. The daily operation is carried out by the elected officers (EXCOM) and the executive secretary.

Activities of the organization are conducted by the administrative committees and the commissions. The administrative committees include the awards and honors, annual meeting, budget and finance, ethics, membership, nominating, and rules committees and the corporate council. There are three commissions: credentials, communications, and professional practice. Under the commission on credentials are the continuing-education and licensure committees. Under the commission on communications are the public relations and publications committees. Under the commission on professional practice are the government affairs, organizational liaison, reimbursement, and standards (therapy and diagnostic) committees. In addition, task groups can be appointed by the chairman or committees. Further information on the various commissions, councils, committees, and task groups can be found in the ACMP bylaws and rules.

5. Selected ACMP accomplishments

The ACMP bylaws state that its objectives are to enhance the quality of the practice of medical physics, engage in professional activities for the benefit of the medical physics community, and promote the continuing competence of the practitioners of medical physics. The ACMP has fulfilled these objectives in many ways, as illustrated by the following selected examples.

By creating a definition for a "qualified medical physicist" in 1986, the ACMP enabled regulatory agencies to designate that certain tasks, such as calibration of diagnostic and therapy machines, were the responsibility of someone trained in medical physics rather than the responsibility of a vendor or serviceman.

The ACMP has been a strong proponent of state licensure of medical physicists and has contributed financially to local groups leading that effort. Licensure for medical physicists is currently available in Texas and Florida and pending in California and New York. Licensure makes it illegal to perform the tasks or duties of a medical physicist without appropriate credentials. This protects both the public and the integrity of our profession.

The ACMP has annual meetings and workshops at which medical physicists can learn about professional issues and develop competency in applications of new technologies. For example, in 1997, at the 14th ACMP Annual Meeting, the topic "Clinical Implementation of 3-D Radiation Therapy" focused on very practical and clinically oriented issues.

The ACMP works cooperatively with outside organizations. The ACMP was responsible for the initiative to form the Trilateral Committee, a group consisting of representatives from the AAPM, the ACMP, and the Commission on Physics of the ACR. The Trilateral Committee coordinates the efforts of the medical physics community that are directed toward common goals. A major effort of this committee took place in June 1997 when the three organizations co-hosted a symposium on professional issues entitled "Adapting to Managed Care."

The ACMP has produced several reports for the clinical medical physicist. Five such reports were produced for diagnostic imaging physics, including operational standards for magnetic resonance imaging and mammography as well as staffing requirements for a diagnostic department (in conjunction with the AAPM). The ACMP and the AAPM collaboratively solicited Abt Associates (Cambridge, MA), which in 1995 produced a report assigning relative value units to the common tasks performed by medical physicists (Abt Associates Inc. 1995). This important information is required by governmental agencies when Medicare and Medicaid reimbursement issues are evaluated. The report also was needed to protect the reimbursement codes designated to physics. More recently, an ACMP task group completed the "Survey of physics resources for radiation oncology special procedures." This document explains the costs required for acquiring and supporting complex special procedures in radiation oncology, such as stereotactic radiosurgery and high-dose-rate brachytherapy (ACMP 1998).

In 1989, the ACMP helped create and continues to sponsor the American Board of Medical Physics, an organization established to address certification issues specific to medical physicists, not just those associated with radiology. It is important to note that this board was established at a time when the American Board of Radiology was unwilling to allow the AAPM to seat three medical physics trustees on its board as it did the other physician disciplines. Although there is talk of a merger of the two boards, it is most important that the resolution between these bodies brings unity to the medical physics community rather than divisiveness.

The ACMP continues to find unique solutions to the needs of the medical physicist. The Board of Chancellors has approved the establishment of a peer-reviewed electronic journal that will emphasize the more clinical, technical, and educational articles that are inappropriate for more scientific medical physics journals. It is expected that this journal will be operational by mid-1999.

6. How to become a member

I was asked by a young physicist at an annual AAPM meeting if being a member of the ACMP would raise his income. After some thought I said "yes," because I believe that the ACMP allows you to develop the skills you will need to have a long and prosperous career. The question is, "When do you want to begin?" Although full membership is reserved for persons who have been in the practice long enough to be certified, there is a provisional membership category that allows less-experienced medical physicists to join the organization. Check the ACMP home page at http://www.acmp.org for membership information and other facts about the ACMP.

7. Conclusion

The ACMP is the only organization created by medical physicists that has the primary charge of addressing the professional concerns of the medical physicist. For 15 years, it has effectively met its objectives and has already had a positive impact on your new profession. Developing scientific and technical skills are paramount at this stage of your career, but you will soon find it necessary to develop managerial and leadership skills. I hope you will consider membership in the ACMP now or very soon, because it is to your benefit to do so.

Acknowledgments

The ACMP would like to thank Kenneth R. Hogstrom, PhD, and John L. Horton, PhD, for offering the ACMP the opportunity to co-sponsor this series on professional issues.

References

Abt Associates Inc. (1995) "The Abt study of medical physicist work values for radiation oncology physics services." Cambridge, MA:Abt Associates Inc.

American College of Medical Physics (1997) "Survey of physics resources for radiation oncology special procedures," ACMP Task Group Report. Reston, VA:ACMP

— (1998) American College of Medical Physics Membership Directory. Reston, VA:ACMP

Grote R (1996) Beyond technology: Finding professional success through personal competence. Presented at the 13th Annual ACMP Meeting, Montreal, Canada

Walter H. Grant III, PhD

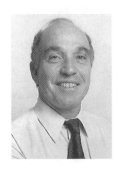

Walter H. Grant III received his PhD in Experimental Nuclear Structure Physics from Tulane University, New Orleans, LA in 1969. He received his training in medical physics as an Advanced Senior Fellow in medical physics at The University of Texas M. D. Anderson Hospital and Tumor Institute (now The University of Texas M. D. Anderson Cancer Center) in Houston, TX from 1969 to 1970. Dr. Grant worked on the staff of M. D. Anderson Cancer Center's Department of Physics from 1970 to 1978, reaching the ranks of Associate Physicist and Assistant Professor of Biophysics. During that term, Dr. Grant also served as Associate Director of the institution's Radiological Physics Center from 1971 to 1975. From 1978 to 1981, Dr. Grant was Physicist for Gulfcoast Oncology Associates, Bayfront Medical Center, St. Petersburg, FL, and from 1981 to the present, he has been president of G III Physics, Inc., St. Petersburg, FL. In 1989, Dr. Grant took his present position of Associate Professor of Radiology, Department of Radiology, Baylor College of Medicine, Houston, TX where he supervises radiotherapy physics services for Baylor's three teaching hospitals: Methodist Hospital, The Veteran's Administration Medical Center, and Ben Taub General Hospital. Dr. Grant's broad range of clinical and professional experience have been valuable in his service to the ACMP, where he has served as a member of the Board of Chancellors, Secretary, newsletter editor, Vice Chairman, Chairman, and Past Chairman. Dr. Grant is a Fellow of the ACMP.

The American College of Radiology: The Organization

Charles A. Kelsey, PhD

Department of Radiology, University of New Mexico, Health Science Center, Albuquerque, NM

Abstract. The American College of Radiology (ACR) is a professional society that works to improve the health of patients and society by maximizing the value of radiology through its active commitment to promoting the technical, scientific, social, and economic aspects of the radiology profession. The ACR accomplishes this by monitoring government actions, promoting accreditation and credentialing, encouraging development of new technology, and helping members adapt to changing times. The ACR is a large organization that is governed by a Council that establishes policy. The Council Steering Committee and the commissions propose policies for consideration by the Council. The Board of Chancellors implements policies established by the Council. The ACR is comprised of approximately 31,800 radiologists, radiation oncologists, and medical physicists in 54 local chapters across the country. Although medical physicists are a small fraction of the total ACR membership, their presence is important, because it lends technical credibility to the ACR. Membership in the ACR strengthens the entire profession of medical physics, improves the economic outlook for medical physicists, and improves communications between medical physicists and local physicians.

1. Introduction

The American College of Radiology (ACR) works to improve the practice of radiology through its active commitment to promoting the technical, scientific, social, and economic aspects of the radiology profession. The ACR accomplishes this by monitoring government actions, promoting accreditation and credentialing, encouraging development of new technology, and helping members adapt to changing times. Membership in the ACR strengthens the entire profession of medical physics, improves the economic outlook for medical physicists, and improves communications between medical physicists and local physicians.

As members of the ACR, medical physicists can impact the economic aspects of their profession by constantly monitoring the rules and regulations promulgated by third-party payers and government entities. Although medical physicists represent only a small fraction of the total ACR membership, their presence lends technical credibility to the ACR. Also, each individual membership by medical physicists in the ACR increases the representation of medical physics both at the local chapter level and at the Council level.

This chapter describes what the ACR is, what it does, how it operates, and the advantages of ACR membership to a medical physicist.

2. What is the ACR?

The ACR is a professional society comprised of approximately 31,800 radiologists, radiation oncologists, and medical physicists in 54 local chapters across the country.

There are two categories of ACR membership: full and associate. To be eligible for full membership, an individual must be a practicing radiologist, radiation oncologist, or medical physicist who is certified by the American Board of Radiology (ABR). Practicing radiologists, radiation oncologists, and medical physicists who are not certified by the ABR may apply for associate membership. The only difference between the two categories is that associate members cannot hold office or chair commissions. Every ACR member belongs to one of the 54 local chapters, which represent each of the 50 states, the District of Columbia, Puerto Rico, Canada, and CARROS (Council of Affiliated Regional Radiation Oncology Societies).

3. What does the ACR do?

The ACR works to improve the health of patients and society by maximizing the value of radiology and radiologists by advancing the science of radiology, improving radiological service to the patient, studying the socio-economic aspects of the practice of radiology, and encouraging continuing education for radiologists and allied professional fields. The ACR accomplishes this by monitoring government actions, promoting accreditation and credentialing, encouraging development of new technology, and helping members adapt to changing times.

3.1. Monitoring government actions

The ACR monitors government actions through its Commission on Government and Public Relations and through its Government Relations Office, which has a paid staff of nine persons. The ACR is a 501-3C organization, which means that it does not perform activities but does inform and educate government agencies and bodies on issues pertaining to radiology. Recently, the Radiology Advocacy Alliance was formed as an Internal Revenue Code 501C-6 organization to engage in both lobbying and political activities.

3.2. Promoting accreditation and credentialing

The ACR promotes accreditation and credentialing by implementing voluntary accreditation programs, promulgating voluntary standards, and sponsoring the ABR. The ACR develops voluntary standards and voluntary accreditation programs that may lead to more formal accreditation and credentialing programs. In the future, accreditation programs will be tied to insurance coverage, hospital privileges, and reimbursement. An agreement is being discussed between the ACR and the Joint Commission on the Accreditation of Healthcare Organizations (JCAHO) whereby the JCAHO will recognize ACR accreditation standards. With this in place, further documentation or investigation by the JCAHO will not be required for ACR-accredited programs.

3.3. Encouraging development of new technology

The ACR encourages development of new technology through: 1) expert assessment and endorsement of new standards of technology and 2) cooperation with industry. Examples include: 1) developing standards for teleradiology and data compression of medical images and 2) working closely with manufacturers to develop and test new radiological technology.

3.4. Helping members adapt to changing times

The ACR helps members adapt to changing times by providing educational and training courses that address changes in practice, technology, and economics. These courses are held throughout the country and at national meetings.

4. How does the ACR operate?

Figure 1 illustrates the organizational structure of the ACR. The ACR has a paid staff of approximately 230 people. The Council is the governing body of the ACR. The Council includes representatives from the local chapters and representatives from other radiological and physics societies. The Council Steering Committee (CSC) and the commissions propose policies that are considered by the ACR Council. The policies of the Council are expressed as resolutions or standards. For example, there is an ACR standard for the diagnostic medical physics performance monitoring of radiographic and fluoroscopic equipment. There also is an ACR policy on magnetic resonance imaging that requires the existence of a documented quality assurance program that is reviewed at least annually by a qualified medical physicist.

4.1. The ACR organization

4.1.1. The Council. The Council is composed of the 258 councilors representing the 54 local chapters and other national radiology and physics organizations, including one from the American Association of Physicists in Medicine (AAPM) and one from the American College of Medical Physics (ACMP). The Council is apportioned so that each chapter has one councilor for every 100 members. Medical physicists are represented as a chapter and likewise are allocated one councilor for every 100 physicist members. At the 1997 Council Meeting, there were 7 physics councilors in attendance. The Council meets annually at a 4-day conference.

4.1.2. Board of Chancellors. The executive branch of the ACR is the Board of Chancellors. The Board has 25 members and is charged with implementing policies established by the Council. The Board also acts on all administrative issues. The Chairman of the Commission on Medical Physics is a member of the Board of Chancellors.

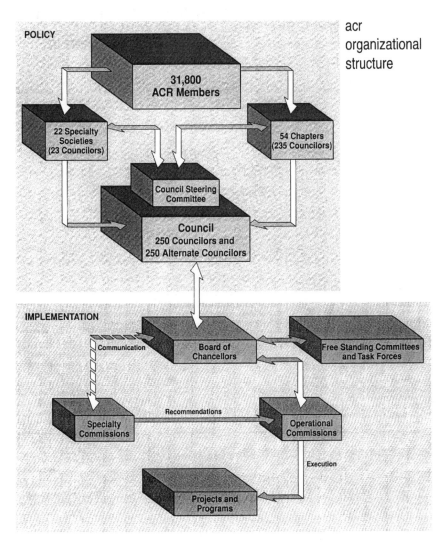

Figure 1. A block diagram showing the organizational structure of the American College of Radiology. Reprinted with permission of the American College of Radiology.

4.1.3. ACR commissions. The ACR commissions and committees assist in the implementation of the policies of the college through their numerous programs and services. There are two types of commissions in the ACR: operational and specialty. The Operational Commissions deal with specific areas of concern and refer issues directly to the Board of Chancellors for consideration. Table 1 lists the ACR Operational Commissions. The Specialty Commissions, which include the Commission on Medical Physics, represent the radiology subspecialties and communicate the needs of the subspecialties to the Board of Chancellors and Operational Commissions. The Specialty Commissions are listed in Table 2.

Horizontal integration between the commissions is accomplished by a parallel committee structure. Every Specialty Commission includes a member from the corresponding Operational Commission. For example, the Specialty Commission on Medical Physics has the following committees: 1) human resources, 2) research and technology assessment, 3) standards and accreditation, 4) government and public relations, 5) economics, and 6) education.

Table 1. ACR Operational Commissions	Table 2. ACR Specialty Commissions
Research and Technology Assessment Standards and Accreditation Economics Education Government and Public Relations Human Resources	Neuroradiology and Magnetic Resonance Medical Physics Radiation Oncology Ultrasound General and Pediatrics Interventional and Cardiovascular Nuclear Medicine

4.1.4. The Council Steering Committee. The CSC has 19 members, one of which is a medical physicist. The CSC was established to handle questions that arise when the Council is not in session. For example, during an out-of-session period, the CSC and the Board of Chancellors recognized that the ACR should take a position regarding teleradiology. They charged the Commission on Standards and Accreditation to develop a standard on teleradiology that could be considered by the Council at its next meeting.

4.2. Accreditation and credentialing

One ACR goal is to have voluntary accreditation programs become so widely accepted that federal legislation is not required. This did not happen in the case with mammography. The ACR voluntary mammography accreditation program was taken over by the Mammography Quality Standard Act (MQSA), which now has the force of law. Early in the development of the voluntary mammography accreditation program, discussions centered on monitoring the technical characteristics of mammography units. There was concern that the requirement that the units be inspected annually by a qualified medical physicist (QMP) could not be met because there were not enough QMPs. ACR standards define a QMP as an individual who is competent to practice independently in one or more of the medical physics subfields. The ACR considers that certification and continuing education in the appropriate subfield or subfields demonstrate competency to practice one or more of the subfields of medical physics and to be deemed a QMP. The ACR recommends that practicing medical physicists be certified in the appropriate subfields by the ABR.

In 1985, the ACR sponsored a study headed by medical physicist member Lawrence Rothenberg to determine whether there were enough QMPs in practice. The survey was completed before the final standards were written, and it demonstrated that there was a sufficient number of QMPs available for practice. The value of services provided by QMPs was recognized by the inclusion of annual QMP surveys in the voluntary accreditation program. That requirement was also carried over into the federal MQSA regulations. There are now ACR-accredited programs for stereotactic breast biopsy, radiation oncology, and ultrasound. Accreditation programs currently under development include programs in chest radiography, nuclear medicine, interventional procedures, and ultrasonic-guided breast biopsies. The ACR is working on an umbrella accreditation program that will encompass multiple modalities.

The ACR monitors the interpretation of regulations established by the federal government, health maintenance organizations, and third-party payers. Some medical physicists might be tempted to ask, "Who cares?" But consider this question: Is it correct to bill a patient for both continuing medical physics consultation (77336) and special medical physics consultation (77370)? The original position of the third-party payers was, "No, never!" They felt the two charges should be bundled together and that only the lower charge should be billed. After negotiations with the ACR, a compromise was reached as an interim solution. The compromise was that the charge should reflect how billing is processed. A 77336 is a weekly charge and can be billed anytime during the week. If it is billed on the same day that a 77370 charge is billed, the two charges will be bundled, and only one (the lower) will be allowed. If the two charges are billed on separate days, they will not be bundled, and both will be allowed. The ACR also took a position in readjusting the 77295 charge for three-dimensional simulation. Some payers required that the treatment beams be noncoplanar in order for the three-dimensional simulation charge to be allowed. After negotiations with the ACR, payers now agree that if certain conditions are met, 77295 will be covered, even if the treatment beams are coplanar.

4.3. ACR standards

Why should anyone care what the standards say? Because in many cases, standards define the level and extent of training and experience required to perform some radiographic testing and evaluation procedures. Interpretation of standards can influence the economics of medical physics. How much training and experience is required to do what? Who should calibrate an x-ray machine—a service engineer, a dosimetrist, a radiation therapist, or a QMP? And even more important, who decides? The answer to the latter question, of course, is the organizations that pay the bills, and generally, they always select the least-expensive choice, unless there is a strong reason to do otherwise. Cost cutters will always look for reasons to reject charges and to use the least-expensive personnel to perform a task.

This is the purpose of standards, and needless to say, there can only be one standard regarding a specific topic or there is no standard. Standards are designed to ensure that the patient receives quality radiology care. Standards cover all aspects of the examination or treatment, including the training, experience, and qualifications of the personnel involved. In addition to the content of the standard, the organization promulgating the standard also is an important factor. If the AAPM or the ACMP states that calibrations of radiation-producing machines should be performed by a QMP, it might be interpreted as a self-serving endorsement by a group of medical physicists. On the other hand, if the ACR, speaking for all professionals involved in radiation-producing health care fields, makes the same statement, it likely would be perceived as an unbiased attempt of a group of experts to obtain the best-quality patient care. When the ACR speaks on behalf of medical physicists, it is not perceived as self-serving, because its medical physicist members are a small fraction of an extremely large medical organization. Medical physicist members are a very important part of the ACR, not only because of the physics knowledge they bring to the organization, but also because the ACR is the only medical organization with a spectrum of members dedicated to ensuring the safe and efficacious use of radiation for patients, staff, and the public.

An important ACR standard currently under development is that radiographic and fluoroscopic equipment should be evaluated by a diagnostic medical physicist. Although the JCAHO requires annual evaluation of radiographic and fluoroscopic equipment, there is no statement establishing who should perform the evaluation. Therefore, many institutions with service contracts would like their service engineers to perform these evaluations. However, should the JCAHO recognize ACR standards, an ACR standard that specifies that a QMP perform these evaluations will eliminate this concern.

4.4. The ACR strategic plan

The ACR has a strategic plan that is based on its view of the future. The plan consists of nine points that are modified here to focus on future effects on medical physics.

1. Legislation and regulations will increase, with many groups trying to influence laws and regulations. The ACR has nine full-time staff members who monitor legislation and regulations. They provide information to legislators and regulators to ensure that radiology and medical physics receive fair and equitable treatment in future laws and regulations. The ACR has demonstrated in the past that it has an effective working relationship with third-party payers and in many cases can modify proposed legislation or regulations during their development by educating all parties. The ACR staff depends on input from the medical physics community to respond to federal and state laws and regulations.

2. Governmental power will shift from a federal to a state level. Local chapters will become even more important in ensuring that medical physics is treated fairly and not lost in the maelstrom of managed care. One disturbing aspect of the new health care models is that the states look to each other for precedents. Thus, a decision in Utah may influence the acceptance of medical physics charges in many other states. For this reason, careful monitoring of local third-party-payer decisions is extremely important.

3. Medical Physicists will be asked to do more work for less pay. This statement describes the future for all health care workers. The ACR strongly supports increased efficiency in all aspects of health care, but it is firmly opposed to attempts to reduce costs at the expense of lowering the quality of health care.

4. Patients and third-party payers will demand quality medical care. A corollary of this demand is that the medical physics community must develop ways to measure the quality of medical physics services. A zero error rate is not an indication of quality medical physics services. Instead, we must define who our customers are, decide what they want and what they need (which may not be the same), and develop methods to quantify the quality of our services. That these are difficult questions does not lessen their importance.

5. There will be an attempt at turf encroachment. Whether by radiation therapists, dosimetrists, health physicists, service engineers, or other individuals with some technical training, there will be assaults on the traditional medical physics turf. However, these individuals do not have the background, training, or experience of a QMP. Replacing QMPs with less-qualified, lower-cost workers can be prevented by providing superior, cost-effective services; developing standards to ensure quality medical physics services; or placing really big bear traps at the edges of our turf.

6. New technologies will be developed, and these new technologies will lead to new turf battles. The only way to stay abreast of new technologies and the changes brought by them is through continuing education. It is the responsibility of medical physicists to continually update their education and skills. The ACR standard on continuing education calls for earning 60 continuing-education credits over a 3-year period. The AAPM program on Remotely Directed Continuing Education provides an opportunity to obtain continuing-education credits over the Internet. This program and others are accredited by the Commission on Accreditation of Medical Physics Education Programs, Inc., which is jointly sponsored by the ACR, the AAPM, and the ACMP.

7. The low-cost approach will probably prevail. Complicated radiation therapy treatment plans with little or no clinical advantage will have to be dropped in favor of standard treatment approaches.

8. Other professional societies will see medical physicists as competitors. We cannot do anything about other societies, but cooperation between the various medical physics societies is essential for the long-term wellbeing of medical physics. Indeed, such cooperation is fostered by continuous communications between the organizations and regular meetings of the Trilateral Committee, a group consisting of representatives from the AAPM, the ACMP, and the ACR Commission on Physics.

9. The public does not know much about medical physics and probably cares even less. A continual effort to educate the public may help define what medical physics is and what we do. Without a strong effort to do so, medical physics services will be driven by price rather than quality.

4.5. The ACR budget

The ACR's nearly $30 million budget is divided to ensure the effective implementation of its charges. About one-third of the income comes from member dues, one-third from the sale of services, and one-third from grants and contracts. National membership dues are $150 per year; chapter dues are additional. Chapter dues for physicists vary from state to state, but most are less than $75 per year.

5. Advantages of ACR membership

Membership in the ACR strengthens the entire profession of medical physics, improves the economic outlook for medical physicists, and improves communications between medical physicists and local physicians. Each individual membership in ACR increases the representation of medical physics both at the local chapter level and at the council level. This means that medical physicists have a greater voice in the development of standards that impact their profession.

As members in the ACR, medical physicists can impact the economic aspects of their profession by constantly monitoring the rules and regulations promulgated by third-party payers and government entities. ACR medical physicists serve on both the Specialty Carrier Advisory Committee, the Coding and Nomenclature Committee, and the Managed Care Committee. These committees monitor the actions of third-party payers and often can modify regulations proposed by the insurance carriers and government agencies before they become policy or law. These behind-the-scenes activities require significant time and dedication on the part of ACR medical physics members; however, such efforts have proven effective in protecting medical physics interests with regard to Current Procedural Terminology (CPT) coding.

Medical physicists are most influential when they participate in the ACR committee structure. However, all ACR medical physicist members help to improve the practice of their profession as well as their own economic wellbeing by increasing their representation in the organization. Members count, and every additional 100 members adds one more medical physicist at the Council meeting.

6. Conclusion

The ACR is an extremely large organization that is governed by a Council, that establishes policy administered by the Board of Chancellors, and that proposes policy to the Council and then implements it once it is established. Although medical physicists are a small fraction of the total ACR membership, their presence is important, because it lends technical credibility to the ACR. Membership in the ACR also provides benefits different than other medical physics-based organizations. The ACR has a professional staff that effectively monitors the actions of third-party payers and advances the professional interests of clinical medical physicists.

Acknowledgments

I wish to thank Robert Breden, Robert Heartland, James Hevezi, Ken Hogstrom, Geoff Ibbott, Richard Lane, Richard Morin, Brad Short, Donald Tolbert, John Trueblood, and David Vassy for their comments and suggestions. Their advice was invaluable. Any errors or omissions in this work are mine, because I did not listen well enough.

References

American College of Radiology (1998) American College of Radiology Resource Guide. Reston, VA: ACR

American Medical Association (1997) Current Procedural Terminology. Chicago, IL: AMA

Charles A. Kelsey, PhD

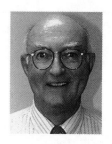

Charles Kelsey received his PhD in Physics from Notre Dame University in 1962. Subsequently (1962 to 1964), Dr. Kelsey trained in medical physics as a postdoctoral fellow at the University of Wisconsin. In 1964, Dr. Kelsey joined the faculty at the University of Wisconsin, where he achieved the rank of Professor of Radiology in 1971. In 1975, Dr. Kelsey joined the University of New Mexico as Chief of Biomedical Physics in the Department of Radiology at the Cancer Research and Treatment Center. In 1989, Dr. Kelsey relinquished that post to concentrate his efforts in diagnostic imaging; he currently serves as Professor of Radiology. Dr. Kelsey has published over 128 peer-reviewed scientific articles and is well known for his research in receiver operating characteristics analysis for diagnostic imaging. Dr. Kelsey is also dedicated to teaching residents and has authored four books. His active involvement in professional societies is evidenced by his being named a Fellow of the AAPM and ACR. Dr. Kelsey has served and chaired the AAPM Radiation Protection Committee since 1992 and the ACR Physics Committee on Research and Technology Assessment since 1992. He has also served as the Vice Chair of the ACR Commission on Medical Physics.

Professional Credentials

Medical Physics Certification: American Board of Radiology and American Board of Medical Physics

James A. Purdy, PhD

Radiation Oncology Center, Mallinckrodt Institute of Radiology, Washington University School of Medicine, St. Louis, MO

Abstract. Obtaining certification in a subspecialty of medical physics is an important step in the career of a clinical medical physicist. The two boards that administer such certification in the United States are the American Board of Radiology and the American Board of Medical Physics. Thus, medical physicists of all ages and in all clinical physics specialties have ample resources to support their certification endeavors. A certification board evaluates the qualifications of voluntary candidates who request examination for certification in a specific medical physics subspecialty; arranges, controls, and conducts examinations to test the competence of candidates seeking certification; grants and issues certificates in the various medical physics subspecialties to qualified applicants; and maintains and makes available to the medical and lay communities a registry of certified medical physicists. This chapter reviews the historical development of these two boards, the certification process conducted by each of the boards, and current issues facing young medical physicists regarding certification.

1. Introduction

The need for credentialing of clinical medical physicists was recognized early in this century and has led to the formation of certification boards for clinical medical physicists. Presently, two boards, the American Board of Radiology (ABR) and the American Board of Medical Physics (ABMP), certify medical physicists in the United States.

A certification board evaluates the qualifications of voluntary candidates who request examination for certification in a specific medical physics subspecialty; arranges, controls, and conducts examinations to test the competence of candidates seeking certification; grants and issues certificates in the various medical physics subspecialties to qualified applicants; and maintains and makes available to the medical and lay communities a registry of certified medical physicists.

With regard to credentialing, the medical physics profession also has embraced the concept of special accreditation of medical physics education and training programs. The Commission on Accreditation of Medical Physics Education Programs, Inc. (CAMPEP) offers accreditation of medical physics advanced-degree and residency programs. CAMPEP is sponsored by the American Association of Physicists in Medicine (AAPM), the American College of Medical Physics (ACMP), and the American College of Radiology (ACR). A graduate-education program in medical physics that is accredited by CAMPEP is recognized as one that conforms to standards that should result in its graduates being qualified for more specialized training or professional practice in clinical medical physics. Although graduation from a medical physics residency program accredited by CAMPEP does not guarantee certification, individuals who successfully complete a CAMPEP residency program should be adequately prepared for the certification examination.

In addition to training-program accreditation and certification of the individual physicist, licensure is recognized as another means to credential clinical medical physicists to ensure that the profession is practiced by competent individuals. The AAPM and ACMP currently support efforts to obtain licensure of medical physicists at the state level; however, only two states, Texas and Florida, have passed legislation requiring licensure of medical physicists. One of the prerequisites for licensure is passing a board certification examination that evaluates competency or an equivalent examination administered by the state.

Until recently, most physicists entering the field of clinical medical physics had no choice but to learn on the job, working under practitioners who were experienced but self-taught. Although academic degree programs (accredited and nonaccredited) existed for medical physicists, there was no organized, standardized clinical training. As a result, a very serious problem existed with regard to ensuring adequate qualifications and competence of medical physicists when they were hired to provide clinical services. Unfortunately, medical physicists are quite often hired on the basis of their academic degrees, with the assumption that the degree programs provide the requisite clinical physics training. However, the clinical physics training component of these programs is either inadequate or nonexistent.

The AAPM recognized this problem and in 1990 published a comprehensive document describing the essential elements of residency training for medical physicists (American Association of Physicists in Medicine 1990). The document established the educational and administrative requirements for a hospital-based physics residency training program patterned after medical residency programs. To date, only a few medical physics residency programs are available in the United States, and only one is thus far accredited by CAMPEP. This situation will likely change rapidly over the next few years. These changes should produce an infrastructure that will provide a formalized clinical medical physics career path. This career path will entail: 1) graduation from an accredited medical physics advanced-degree program, 2) completion of an accredited medical physics residency program, 3) certification in a specific medical physics subspecialty, and 4) licensing to practice that subspecialty. I believe that the medical physics profession already is moving in this direction and that this goal is achievable over the next 10 years.

Other chapters in this book will deal directly with licensing, but this chapter will focus on medical physics certification, reviewing the development of the ABR and ABMP, the certification processes, and the certification issues now facing young medical physicists.

2. The history of the development of the ABR and the ABMP

Considerable details on the development of the ABR can be found in articles by Taylor (1981) and Krohmer (1995); details of the development of the ABMP can be found in the article by Suntharalingam (1995). In addition, the text by Gagliardi and Almond (1996) provides additional information about these organizations, including details about their development. Information from these sources is summarized here in a more integrated form so you might better appreciate the events that led to the establishment of the two medical physics certification boards.

2.1. The Radiological Society of North America

The first effort that led to certification of clinical medical physicists can be traced to the Radiological Society of North America (RSNA) Standardization Committee, which was formed in 1925 (Taylor 1981). By 1934, the radiology field had matured, and the need for a mechanism by which a physicist could be certified as competent to perform clinical applications of radiation was recognized. That year, the Standardization Committee produced the draft of a report recommending that a registry of x-ray physicists be established. A portion of that report is reproduced here from the text by Taylor (1981).

> "There was a lengthy discussion on the subject of the calibration of X-ray machines in situ. There has been much abuse along such lines, particularly by people unqualified to make such calibrations. There has been open criticism of the physicist by the physician for frequently offering advice regarding the utilization of radiation in treatment, even to the extent of suggesting proper dosages. Complaint has also been made against manufacturers' agents where it has been alleged that improper calibrations have been given for sales purposes. It was decided, therefore, to set up a Registry of X-Ray Physicists, listing physicists suitably qualified to make calibrations of X-ray machines. It is felt that this will offer protection both to the physician and physicist. It was agreed that a "Registered X-Ray Physicist" should meet the following requirements:
>
> (1) Be a recognized physicist.
> (2) Show a reasonable working knowledge of physics in the radiology field.
> (3) Be familiar with classical X-ray theory.
> (4) Appear before a selected board for examination if deemed advisable by that board.
> (5) Use only such dosage instruments as are approved by the Committee and tested by a recognized testing laboratory. (For example, National Bureau of Standards, Cleveland Clinic, Memorial Hospital, National Research Council of Canada, Temple University Hospital.)
> (6) Agree not to give out any medical information.
> (7) Not be directly employed by any X-ray equipment manufacturer, agent, or distributor."

The members of the RSNA Standardization Committee's first Examining Board were Otto Glasser, PhD; Giacomo Failla, DSc; Lauriston S. Taylor, DSc; and Robert R. Newell, MD (Taylor 1981). In the certification process, a single board member examined an applicant and prepared a written report with recommendations, which was then submitted to the other members of the board for final action. The seriousness of this process can be appreciated by the fact that all papers relating to an applicant and the subsequent certification were filed at the National Bureau of Standards. By the end of 1936, 15 physicists had been certified by this process (Krohmer 1995).

2.2. The American Board of Radiology

Certification of physicians practicing radiology also was an important issue during this time period. Five radiological societies, the American Roentgen Ray Society, the RSNA, the American Radium Society, the ACR, and the Section on Radiology of the American Medical Association had begun working together to address this matter, and their efforts led to the founding of the ABR, which was officially incorporated in 1934 (Gagliardi and Almond 1996). Thus, in 1936, two important radiology credentialing bodies existed: the ABR for certification of physicians practicing radiology and the RSNA Standardization Committee for certification of clinical medical physicists working in radiology.

Within just a few years, efforts were made to consolidate the certification efforts and have the ABR assume responsibility for certification of clinical medical physicists involved in radiology practice (Gagliardi and Almond 1996). However, it was not until 1947 that this consolidation of certification processes was accomplished, when Dr. Taylor was informed by letter that the ABR had decided to begin certifying physicists. Details were quickly worked out, and three physicists (Drs. Taylor and Glasser and Edith H. Quimby) were elected (from a slate of six nominees selected by the ABR Trustees) by the registered x-ray physicists at that time to serve as the Examining Board for Medical Physicists. In addition, U. V. Portmann, MD, also was appointed by the ABR to serve on the Examining Board. Dr. Taylor, however, withdrew from the Examining Board. Dr. Failla was then named but also declined. The vacancy was finally filled when Marvin M. D. Williams, PhD, agreed to assume the position. From these actions, one could infer that there was some dissatisfaction in this turn of events, but it was not well documented. Dr. Taylor has reported that some of the radiological physicists at that time were unhappy with the decision to have the ABR certify physicists. They felt alienated because critical actions had been taken without their knowledge (Taylor 1981).

The first formal ABR certification examination of medical physicists was held in Atlantic City, NJ, in June 1949, and included five candidates (Krohmer 1995). That examination involved an oral test only; but the process was changed immediately to require the applicant to submit specific written reports, depending on the medical physics subspecialty, that were reviewed before the applicant was admitted to the oral examination. This requirement remained in effect until 1975, when these reports were replaced by a written examination that included didactic radiological physics questions as well as clinically oriented questions (Krohmer 1995). The oral examination also was changed to focus mainly on equipment and procedures used in everyday radiological physics practice. This format has essentially remained unchanged to the present day (Krohmer 1995). However, the ABR has decided that a restructuring of the examination for physicists is needed and that it should involve changes in all parts of the written and oral examination (American Board of Radiology 1997a). Details of these changes were not available at the time of this writing.

Another important issue for medical physicists was physics representation on the ABR certifying board. In 1949, at the time of the first ABR examination of physicists, the three physicists on the Examining Board for Physicists met with the ABR trustees only when the results of the physicists' examinations were being discussed and acted on (Krohmer 1995). This did not change for almost 20 years when, in 1968, Dr. Williams began attending all meetings of the ABR trustees; but, as reported by Krohmer (1995), Dr. Williams participated with "voice only and not vote." Dr. Williams attended the trustee meetings in this capacity until 1972, when he was succeeded by Jack Krohmer, PhD.

2.3 The American Board of Medical Physics

It was also in 1972 that the need for a separate, independent certification board for medical physicists in the United States was first publicly raised. The idea was presented at the AAPM annual meeting (Suntharalingam 1995). Over the next decade, this matter continued to be informally debated within the medical physics community, particularly during the initial years of the ACMP. In 1984, an ACMP task group was appointed specifically to study the need for a separate, independent board in the United States that was governed by medical physicists and focused on the certification of medical physicists (Suntharalingam 1995). In 1985, the task group's recommendations prompted the ACMP to proceed with the establishment of an American Board of Medical Physics that would offer to medical physicists "peer certification in the physical aspects of radiation therapy, diagnostic radiology and nuclear medicine, as well as other areas of medical physics" (Suntharalingam 1995).

During this same period, the AAPM sought to become an official sponsoring organization of the ABR. In 1979, the ABR had approved the appointment of an official physics trustee to the board, and although the AAPM was not approved as a sponsoring society, it was asked to name three individuals as nominees for this position. The ABR trustees elected Dr. Krohmer, who had been serving in a "voice only and not vote" capacity since 1972. Dr. Krohmer officially started a 6-year term as the ABR physics trustee on January 1, 1981, and subsequently was reelected for a second 6-year term that started January 1, 1987.

In 1982, the AAPM stepped up its efforts to become an official sponsoring organization of the ABR and thus have three physics trustees as representatives, similar to the other sponsoring organizations. However, this proved to be a very difficult task and again led to disenchantment with the ABR by some medical physicists. In 1988, a compromise was finally reached among the AAPM leadership, the ABR, and sponsoring ABR societies in which the AAPM became an official ABR-sponsoring organization with the restriction that it would have only one trustee. Once again, however, this left some medical physicists upset, because they believed that the one trustee, compared with the three trustees the other sponsoring organizations were allowed, inferred "second-class citizenship" for the AAPM and, more importantly, for the medical physics profession. Efforts continued, however, and in 1994, the ABR finally approved three physics trustees. Again, however, some restrictions were imposed; only one trustee in each of three subspecialties was allowed: therapeutic radiological physics, diagnostic radiological physics, and medical nuclear physics, although most clinical medical physicists involved in radiology were radiation oncology physicists. These events are somewhat telling in that the real struggle for AAPM sponsorship may have focused more on conflict between diagnostic radiology physicians and radiation oncology physicians than on a medical physics issue.

In 1986, a constituting panel was organized by the ACMP to develop guidelines for establishment of the new ABMP. Nine professional societies, including the AAPM, the American Society of Therapeutic Radiology and Oncology (ASTRO), and the RSNA, appointed official representatives to the panel and thus had an opportunity, at an early stage, for direct involvement in shaping policy of this new board (Suntharalingam 1995). In 1987, the ACMP became the first sponsoring organization of the ABMP and appointed the first six medical physicists to the board of directors. They were Robert Gorson, MS; Edward Nickoloff, DSc; Colin Orton, PhD; Bhudatt Paliwal, PhD; James Purdy, PhD; and Edward Sternick, PhD. The ABMP was incorporated in the state of Massachusetts as an independent not-for-profit corporation in July 1988 with Dr. Sternick as chairman of the board and Dr. Purdy as vice chairman.

While the ABMP certification-by-examination process was being developed, an inaugural ABMP certification without examination was offered to practicing clinical medical physicists who were able to meet certain strict requirements. These requirements included having been previously certified by a recognized board (e.g., the ABR, the American Board of Health Physics, or the Canadian College of Medical Physics); having had at least 10 years of full-time equivalent experience in clinical medical physics; and having participated in a significant number of documented, formal, continuing medical physics education activities (Suntharalingam 1995). A total of 321 senior clinical medical physicists were awarded ABMP inaugural certification, which ended in December 1990. This relatively large number of senior clinical medical physicists, most of whom were previously certified by the ABR, was viewed as strong support for the ABMP certification program. The first ABMP written certification examination was given in July 1989, and the first oral examination was given in 1990. The number of medical physicists who have received certification by the ABMP after successfully completing the three-part examination process is 176;

thus, a total of 497 medical physicists had been certified by the ABMP as of June 1997, compared with 1831 certified by the ABR as of 1997.

ABMP certification has been officially recognized by regulatory bodies such as the United States Nuclear Regulatory Commission and State Radiation Control agencies (Suntharalingam 1995). In addition, the United States Food and Drug Administration has recognized ABMP certification in diagnostic imaging physics as an acceptable qualification of medical physicists involved in implementing the Mammography Quality Standards Act of 1992 (Suntharalingam 1995). ASTRO and RSNA recognize ABMP certification of medical physicists for membership eligibility criteria. Also, all current definitions of a "qualified medical physicist" that are used by several organizations, including the AAPM and ACMP, and that are written into official documents recognize ABMP certification (Suntharalingam 1995).

The number of medical physicists seeking board certification increased dramatically during the 1990s as these clinicians have become much more cognizant of the importance of credentialing in their profession. This increase is illustrated in Figure 1, which shows the number of candidates who took the ABR and the ABMP oral examinations from 1993 to 1997 (American Board of Radiology 1997b; Suntharalingam 1995; Khan, personal communication, 1997).

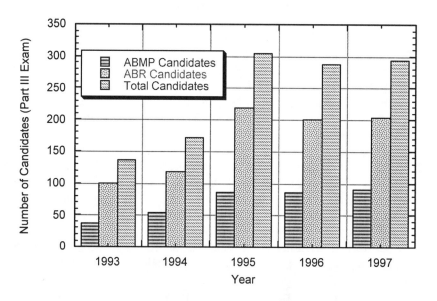

Figure 1. Number of candidates examined by the ABMP and the ABR from 1993 to 1997.

This historical review clearly shows that medical physics board certification has been an evolutionary process, a process that will surely continue to change to meet the needs of all clinical medical physicists. Clinical medical physicists now have two highly effective boards that provide the opportunity to obtain certification. Thus, the practice of medical physicists providing clinical physics services without board certification can no longer be defended and should not be allowed to continue into the 21st century.

3.   The certification process

The ABR currently provides for certification by examination, in the following specialties: 1) therapeutic radiological physics; 2) diagnostic radiological physics; 3) medical nuclear physics; and 4) radiological physics, which includes therapeutic radiological physics, diagnostic radiological physics, and medical nuclear physics (including radiation safety).   The ABMP currently provides for certification by examination in the following specialties: 1) radiation oncology physics, 2) diagnostic imaging physics, 3) medical health physics, and 4) hyperthermia physics.   The ABMP will begin providing certification in magnetic resonance imaging (MRI) in 1998, when the first MRI written examination will be offered; this will be followed by the first MRI oral examination in 1999.

The ABR and the ABMP use written and oral examinations and both must be passed to obtain medical physics certification. In both board processes, the written examinations are divided into two distinct tests.   Part I is a general physics examination containing questions about basic physics, imaging physics, radiation oncology physics, nuclear medicine physics, and some clinical concepts. In Part I of the ABR examination, the questions on the clinical aspects of radiologic physics are actually graded as a separate portion of the test. The Part II written examination for both boards is designed to test the competence of the candidate in a subspecialty area of medical physics, such as radiation oncology physics. More details on the categories and examples of the types of questions asked are available on the ABR and the ABMP World Wide Web sites (www.theabr.org and www.acmp.org, respectively).

After successfully passing the prerequisite Part I and Part II written examinations, candidates are required by both boards to pass an oral examination (Part III) to complete the certification process. The purpose of the oral examination is to ensure that the candidate has sufficient clinical experience and can demonstrate proper responses to simulated clinical situations.

The ABMP oral examination is approximately 2 hours long. Each candidate is examined by a panel of three or four examiners, one of whom serves as the chairman. The examination covers the following eight subject categories with each examiner responsible for leading the questioning in two or three categories: 1) treatment machines/simulators, 2) radiation measurements/detectors, 3) clinical treatment planning, photon-beam therapy, 4) clinical treatment planning, electron-beam therapy, 5) brachytherapy, 6) radiation safety/hazards, 7) special techniques, and 8) treatment-planning computer systems. Each examiner assigns a score for each category examined. The candidate must receive a passing score from at least all but one examiner in each category in order to pass.

In the ABR oral examination, which lasts approximately 3 hours, the candidate is tested by six physics examiners, one-on-one, for 30 minutes each. During each session, the examiner asks one question from each of the following categories: 1) design of radiation installations, 2) calibration of radiation equipment, 3) radiation hazard control, 4) radiation dosage, and 5) equipment. Each examiner assigns a score to the response to each question. The final score in a particular category is the average of the six scores assigned by the six examiners. When all six sessions are complete, the candidate's performance is evaluated by the full panel of examiners.

It should be noted that the ABMP oral examination process utilizes practicing medical physicists who are ABMP or ABR certified in the subspecialty field in which a candidate is being examined. However, the ABR requires medical physicists to be certified by the ABR. Also, the ABR allows medical physicists certified in radiological physics to serve as examiners for an oral examination in a subspecialty field, even if they are not currently working in that subspecialty.

Candidates who fail in two or more of the five categories of the ABR oral examination must repeat the entire oral examination. Candidates who fail in only one category are awarded a conditional pass, and they must pass an additional oral examination given later in the year to remove the condition. The ABMP also allows for a conditional pass. Candidates who fail in only one or two categories are awarded a conditional pass and must pass an additional oral examination the following year to remove the condition. Candidates who fail three or more of the eight categories must repeat the entire oral examination.

The pass-fail rate varies somewhat. For example, a total of 204 candidates took the 1997 ABR oral examination in one or more of the subspecialties of radiological physics: 64.2% passed, 14.2% conditionally passed, and 21.6% failed (American Board of Radiology 1997b). In the case of the ABMP, a total of 90 candidates took the 1997 oral examination: 44.4% passed, 26.7% conditionally passed, and 28.9% failed (Khan, personal communication, 1997).

The fee structures for the two board-examination processes are different. The ABMP general medical physics (Part I) and subspecialty (Part II) written examinations are $200 each and the oral (Part III) examination is $300, for a total of $700. The ABR has a flat fee of $800.

The minimum educational requirements for admission to the examinations are similar for the two boards: each requires the applicant to have a graduate degree in physics, medical physics, or an appropriate related field from an accredited university. However, the professional-experience requirements differ (Tables 1 and 2). Note that the professional-experience requirements listed for the ABR are for a single subspecialty of medical physics only.

Table 1. ABMP Experience Eligibility Requirements*

- Part I Written Exam (general medical physics)
  - No professional experience required

- Part II Written Exam (subspecialites: radiation oncology physics, diagnostic imaging physics, hyperthermia physics, medical health physics, magnetic resonance imaging physics)
  - Must have received clinical residency training from an accredited program or must have been engaged in the practice of clinical medical physics as a postgraduate under the supervision of a board-certified medical physicist for a minimum period of time preceding the date of the examination as listed below
  - Experience for medical health physics must be obtained as a provider of services in a health care facility

Highest Degree	Years of Experience Required for Part II
MS	4
MS (medical physics)	2
MS (medical physics; accredited)	1
PhD	2
PhD (medical physics)	1
PhD (medical physics; accredited)	1
PhD (accredited clinical residency)	0

- Part III Oral Exam (subspecialties: radiation oncology physics, diagnostic imaging physics, hyperthermia physics, medical health physics, magnetic resonance imaging physics).
  - Must have successfully passed Parts I and II
  - Must have been engaged in the practice of clinical medical physics as a postgraduate for a minimum period of time preceding the date of the examination as listed below
  - Experience for medical health physics must be obtained as a provider of services in a healthcare facility
  - Only one-half of total training years will be credited toward professional experience; applicants from clinical residency programs will receive full credit

Highest Degree	Years of Experience Required for Part III
MS	6
MS (medical physics)	4
MS (medical physics; accredited)	3
PhD	4
PhD (medical physics)	3
PhD (medical physics; accredited)	2
PhD (accredited clinical residency)	1

---

*Summarized from information obtained from the ABMP Web site (www.acmp.org).

Table 2. ABR Experience Eligibility Requirements*

- Part I Written Exam (general medical physics)
  - Beginning in 1998, applicants can take Part I, comprising a general physics section and a clinical section, at any time during their graduate training in an approved program.

- Part II Written Exam (subspecialties: therapeutic radiologic physics, diagnostic radiologic physics, medical nuclear physics)
  - Must have had at least 3 years of full-time active association with an approved department or division of the subspecialty; the experience requirements are discussed in the Essentials document, which can be found on the ABR Web site.
  - Experience requirements must be satisfied by June 30 of the year in which the written examination is taken
  - Experience is deemed to begin no earlier than the candidate's enrollment in an approved program of graduate study

- Part III Oral Exam (subspecialities: therapeutic radiologic physics, diagnostic radiologic physics, medical nuclear physics).
  - Must have successfully passed Parts I and II
  - Must have had at least 3 years of full-time active association with an approved department or division of the subspecialty; the experience requirements are discussed in the Essentials document, which can be found on the ABR Web site

Note: The ABR states that "The 36 months of full-time active association with an approved department(s) or division(s) may be partially acquired by experience associated with graduate study in an approved medical physics program which includes a clinical component. Credit will not be given for experience gained while pursuing an undergraduate degree. Generally not more than half-time credit up to a maximum of 1 year will be credited towards training. Full-time credit will be given for experience gained through approved postgraduate clinical medical physics internship or residency programs and clinical postdoctoral programs. For postdoctoral programs that involve both clinical and research responsibilities, the candidate will receive credit for the clinical component. In the latter case, the candidate's preceptor must confirm the percent of time spent on clinical duties."

Beginning in the year 2000, credit will not be given for extracurricular experience gained before the candidate has attained the master's degree. Until the year 2000, the maximum allowed credit for extracurricular experience is 1 year.

Full-time active association with an approved department or division may be arranged through some other department, such as physics or biophysics, but the work performed by the applicant must be in the appropriate subspecialty of radiologic physics in the approved department or division. The work must be performed under the supervision of a radiologic physicist and/or a radiologic physician. The physicist, physician, or both must be certified by the ABR in the subspecialty in which the applicant claims experience.

---

*Summarized from information obtained from the ABR Web site (www.theabr.org).

The ABR written examinations are typically offered in September, and the ABR oral examinations are offered at the end of May or early June. The ABMP written examinations are offered on the weekend at the start of the AAPM meeting, and the ABMP oral examination is offered during the third or fourth week of April. Information regarding application deadlines for these exams can be found by checking each board's World Wide Web site.

ABMP certification must be renewed every 10 years. Recertification of medical physicists is under consideration by the ABR, and a policy is likely to be adopted in the future.

Physicists considering certification are advised to continue to update the information provided in this chapter by checking each board's Web site.

4. Summary and conclusions

Medical physics certification is an important step in the career of a clinical physicist. As the various medical disciplines in which physicists participate continue to become more clinically complex, the pathway for the clinical physics profession should become more formalized (i.e., graduation from an accredited medical physics degree program followed by clinical physics training in an accredited physics residency program and subsequent board certification). Federal or state licensure will surely follow, thus ensuring that high-quality clinical physics is practiced in clinics throughout the country.

The medical physics community is now served by two certifying boards. For some, this has become a divisive issue, and attempts have recently been made to consolidate certification of medical physicists under a single board. In 1996, the AAPM Board of Directors passed resolutions that endorsed the creation of a Medical Physics Board Certification Council that would exist within the framework of the ABR and consist of representatives from the AAPM, ACMP, ACR Commission on Physics (ACRCOP), and possibly other organizations. An ad hoc committee, which consisted of the AAPM president and representatives of the ABR, ABMP, ACMP, and ACRCOP, was appointed to determine the membership and structure of the Medical Physics Board Certification Council. Considerable effort has been expended, but consolidation does not appear likely anytime soon. It is clear that the AAPM membership consists of large groups of individuals who hold sincere but divergent views regarding clinical medical physics board certification. Some ABR-certified physicists feel strongly that it is important that the medical physicist certification process be recognized by the American Board of Medical Specialties (ABMS). Others feel that this is not important because medical physicists are not physicians and because the ABMS charter is aimed specifically for boards certifying physicians. Currently, the ABMS recognizes the ABR, but the ABMP has not yet applied for such recognition. Some ABMP-certified physicists argue that in the 21st century, areas of medical physics other than radiology and radiation oncology will likely present new opportunities for medical physicists; thus, it is essential that the medical physics certification process not be limited to radiological areas. Other issues that have been raised include: 1) the fact that only potential trustees from a sponsoring organization are nominated (currently such nominations can be accepted or rejected by the board) and 2) the absence of specific reference to medical physics in the ABR name. Unfortunately, in many instances, the debate over these and other issues has become more emotional than rational.

My advice is that clinical medical physicists not yet certified should support both boards. Some will argue that this dual support is a waste of resources; however, I believe that the existence of the two boards has been positive for medical physics certification. Remember that "certification" is the issue of importance not some "ABR versus ABMP" situation. As medical physicists, we should be proud of our over 50 years of working with the ABR in the certification of clinical medical physicists. Likewise, I think we should be proud of the establishment of the ABMP, which offers medical physicists peer certification in the physical aspects of radiation therapy, diagnostic radiology, and nuclear medicine, as well as other areas of medical physics. The important point, I believe, is that there is always likely to be a contingent of medical physicists who would prefer to be certified by a board of their medical physics peers. Similarly, I think there will always be a group of medical physicists who would prefer to be certified by a medical board. I also believe that the existence of competing boards has improved the certification process and helped to increase the medical physics trustee representation in the ABR. Hopefully, reports such as this will foster a spirit of cooperation between the two boards and a commitment to continue to develop a consistent high-quality certification process for medical physicists.

References

American Association of Physicists in Medicine (1990) "Essentials and guidelines for hospital based medical physics residency training programs," AAPM Report No. 36. Woodbury, NY: AIP

American Board of Radiology (1997a) Physics exam restructuring. *ABR Examiner* **2**(1),4

— (1997b) Results of examinations in radiologic physics. *ABR Examiner* **2**(2),10

Gagliardi RA and Almond PR, eds. (1996) A History of the Radiological Sciences: *Radiation Physics*. Reston, VA: Radiology Centennial, Inc.

Krohmer JS (1995) Certification of physicists by the American Board of Radiology. *Medical Physics* **22**,1955-1960

Suntharalingam N (1995) The American Board of Medical Physics. *Medical Physics* **22**,1961-1963

Taylor LS, ed. (1981) "X-ray Measurements and Protection 1913-1964: The role of the National Bureau of Standards and the National Radiological Organizations," NBS Special Publication 625. Washington, DC: NBS

James A. Purdy, PhD

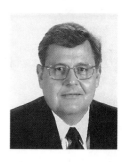

James Purdy received his PhD in Nuclear Physics from The University of Texas at Austin in 1971, which was followed by 1 year of training in medical physics as a postdoctoral fellow in the Department of Physics at The University of Texas M. D. Anderson Hospital and Tumor Institute (now The University of Texas M. D. Anderson Cancer Center) in Houston, TX. In 1973, Dr. Purdy joined the faculty at the Washington University School of Medicine as Instructor in Radiation Physics in Radiology, where he was promoted through the ranks to Professor in 1983. Since 1976, he has served as Chief of the Physics Section, Division of Radiation Oncology, and since 1987, he has served as Associate Director for Quality Assurance of the Radiation Oncology Center. As an academician, Dr. Purdy has authored approximately 200 publications and has established himself as a leader in three-dimensional treatment-planning research. He served on the National Institute of Health Radiation Study Section from 1991 to 1995 and is presently Senior Editor (Physics) for the *International Journal of Radiation Oncology, Biology, Physics*. Dr. Purdy has been a strong supporter of professional medical physics, having served as President of the AAPM and Chairman of the ACMP Board of Chancellors. He has chaired or served on task groups, committees, and boards of directors for several professional societies. He examined for the ABMP from 1989 to1996 and served on the ABR Exam Committee for Radiation Oncology residents from 1987 to 1993. He also served on the ABMP Board of Directors from 1988 to 1992. Dr. Purdy is a Fellow of the AAPM, ACMP, and ACR and has received the AAPM William D. Coolidge Award for Distinguished Contributions to Medical Physics and the ACMP Marvin M. D. Williams Professional Achievement Award, the highest honors bestowed by those societies.

Licensure and Credentialing for Medical Physicists

David L. Goff, PhD

Medical and Radiation Physics, Inc., San Antonio, TX

Abstract. Licensure provides individuals with state-government authorization to practice his or her profession. The professional license establishes minimum requirements for training, experience, and qualifications of the artisan or practitioner and sets standards for the quality of the service to be provided. Licensure minimizes the potential for fraud and for harm to the recipients of a service. For the medical physicist, the benefits of licensure include professional recognition, medical-corporation ownership privilege, and legal protection. At the time of this writing, only two states had achieved licensure: Texas in May 1991 and Florida in June 1995. As of 1995, 449 Texas medical physicists licenses had been granted to residents of the state and 288 to residents of other states. Because of the benefits of licensure for the patient, the public, and the professional medical physicist, we must continue to encourage all states to adopt licensure for medical physicists. Credentialing grants individuals the privilege to practice or perform specified tasks under the supervision of a local, private board. One advantage of credentialing for medical personnel is that rules can be established to handle disputes that arise between the practitioner and the administration of the institution where he or she practices. As our profession matures, we can expect licensure and credentialing for medical physicists to be required as for physicians, dentists, and other health care providers.

1. Introduction

Licensure and credentialing give the qualified medical physicist permission to engage in clinical practice. A license provides state-government authorization; a credential provides institutional authorization. Both types of authorization are aimed at protecting the patient, public, institution, profession, and professional by ensuring that only qualified individuals are allowed to practice medical physics.

This chapter reviews the origins of professional licensure, and it presents the reasons why licensure is advantageous. It provides a brief historical summary of the ongoing quest of medical physicists to secure licensure, including details of the process Texas followed to have its licensure act drafted through the state legislature. The requirements for obtaining a medical physicist license in Texas are outlined. Finally, the various aspects of credentialing for the medical physicist are discussed.

2. Origins of licensure

The precepts of occupational licensing seem to have originated in England in about the 10th century. There, merchants and artisans formed workers guilds through which they assisted each other in times of need. The guilds also protected these workers from the harsh restrictions imposed by the manor lords. The guilds were voluntary associations that tended to monopolize an occupation by enforcing regulations to ensure that workers obtained appropriate training and experience through apprenticeships and journeyman services. Workers who did not meet the guild's requirements were discouraged from performing services offered by members of a guild.

After the collapse of the Roman Empire, the classical curriculum, which was broadened to include languages, logic, mathematics, music, and astronomy, was made available to the public. The demand for teachers grew, and teacher guilds, which later became universities, were formed. The guilds began to establish teaching standards and to demand freedom from church and state authority, thus initiating the concept of academic freedom. This recognized emphasis on knowledge likely aided in the evolution of the Renaissance period. Interestingly, guilds, which are, in effect, precursors to professional licensure, are recognized as major proponents of academic freedom and professional responsibility.

In the United States, the licensing of individuals to practice medicine was first established in Virginia in 1639. By the early 1900s, most states also licensed attorneys, dentists, pharmacists, physicians, and teachers. Now, nearing the end of the 20th century, over 800 occupations and professions are licensed by the individual states. Medical physics is a relatively new profession, but the need for a license to practice within the profession is fast being realized.

3. Reasons for licensing medical physicists

The reasons for requiring a license to practice a profession are very similar to the reasons the early guilds were formed: 1) licensure establishes minimum requirements for training, experience, and qualifications of the artisan or practitioner and 2) licensure sets standards for the quality of the service to be provided. In addition, licensure: 1) establishes professional codes of conduct and ethics, 2) provides a mechanism by which incompetent or unethical practitioners can be removed, and 3) provides a mechanism by which a regulatory authority can identify responsible practitioners; this same mechanism can be used by lay administrators or the public when searching for a capable practitioner.

Another reason why professional licensure should be pursued is because the potential for fraud and harm to patients exists when the practitioner is minimally trained, unskilled, or unscrupulous. In diagnostic imaging, for example, the qualified medical physicist performs and reports the radiation measurements needed for regulatory compliance in the diagnostic x-ray department. If the measurements are incorrect, the patient or the technician may be overexposed to radiation, which could increase their risk for cancer. Incorrect measurements also may result in suboptimal operation of diagnostic equipment, which could result in a false diagnosis leading to undesirable ramifications for both the patient and the physician. Similarly, in radiation therapy, the qualified medical physicist performs and reports radiation measurements needed for regulatory compliance of therapeutic radiation equipment. The medical physicist also controls patient treatment planning and is responsible for ensuring that the levels of radiation prescribed for patient treatment are accurately delivered. Errors such as incorrect machine calibrations or incorrect dosimetry calculations can be harmful for patients and place the institution, the radiation oncologist, and the medical physicist at legal risk. Also, inaccurate safety measurements and calculations or improper safety procedures place the public and health care workers at risk. It should be obvious, but this statement warrants reiteration: The medical physicist's role in radiation therapy usually affects every patient being treated, because we ensure that the dose plan prescribed by the radiation oncologist is indeed delivered by the therapy unit or other sources.

Based on these examples, establishing minimum qualifications and standards of practice for the medical physicist through the licensure process seems reasonable and, indeed, necessary to minimize the potential for fraud and harm to the recipients of our services. Regulatory supervision by state and federal radiation control agencies has limited success in uncovering an improper or fraudulent practitioner, because the inspection intervals are long, the regulatory standards are frequently antiquated and unreflective of current practices, and the typical inspector receives only limited training in the requirements and demands of clinical practice.

Licensure also provides personal benefits for the medical physicist. Being licensed can result in professional recognition, such as inclusion of the medical physicist as a member of the hospital medical staff. Licensure also grants the medical physicist medical-corporation ownership privileges. In California, for example, licensed health personnel can hold minority ownership in medical corporations, allowing the medical physicist to have an equity interest in the professional practice with which he or she is affiliated. Medical-corporation ownership also provides tax benefits for retirement plans and fringe benefits. Licensure also protects the medical physicist against frivolous law suits, because licensure establishes one as a professional, and in most states, tort law forbids bringing suit against a professional without an accompanying affidavit by an expert witness that negligence has occurred (Wright 1991).

4. History of state licensure of medical physicists

In the early 1980s, medical physicists began to intensify their pursuit of licensure. At the first annual meeting of the American College of Medical Physics (ACMP) in 1985, Jim Deye discussed the pros and cons of licensure and strategic issues (Deye 1985), and at the annual meeting of the American Association of Physicists in Medicine (AAPM) in Seattle in 1985, the AAPM Professional Council presented a symposium on licensure. These and other discussions initiated a national interest in establishing a process to obtain state licensure for medical physicists. The ACMP stated its position on licensure in the following resolution, which was adopted on January 31, 1992, in Reston, VA (American College of Medical Physics 1992).

ACMP RESOLUTION

LICENSURE FOR MEDICAL PHYSICISTS

WHEREAS, Patients, members of the public, and health-care workers are entitled to protection of their health and well-being from the harmful effects of excessive amounts of ionizing radiation or the misapplication of ionizing radiation; and

WHEREAS, The practice of Medical Physics is potentially dangerous to patients, members of the public, and health-care workers if performed by persons with insufficient knowledge and training; and

WHEREAS, The privilege of practicing Medical Physics should be entrusted only to those persons who are duly qualified; now, therefore, be it

RESOLVED, That the American College of Medical Physics supports licensure of Medical Physicists in the clinical environment throughout the United States and all its territories.

According to the strategy outlined, state licensure would first be obtained in key states. Texas, Florida, California, and New York were targeted, but efforts were also initiated in Pennsylvania and South Carolina. It was believed that by achieving momentum toward licensure in key states, other states would follow (Mills 1991). At the time of this writing, only two states had achieved licensure: Texas in May 1991 and Florida in June 1995, and the licensure effort in California, although unsuccessful to date, had progressed to the point of only needing the governor's approval. Such efforts will continue until licensure is achieved in all 50 states. To better appreciate the process involved in achieving state licensure as law, I have summarized the Texas licensure effort, with which I am most familiar.

In 1987, the Board of Chancellors of the ACMP funded the formation of the Texas Medical Physics Society (TMPS), a nonprofit corporation established to coordinate the Texas licensure effort and to be a model for other states in their licensure efforts. The first TMPS officers were medical physicists Ann Wright, Michael Mills, Alan Huddleston, and myself; the first corporate board members also were medical physicists Stewart Bushong (chairman), Art Boyer, David Gager, Edward Murphy, Wayne Wiatrowski, and John Horton. A Practice Act was drafted and distributed to qualified parties for review. Later, in 1988, other medical physics organizations were asked to support the licensure effort through formal endorsement resolutions and funding. Dues from over 40 TMPS members and contributions from the ACMP; the New York, Southwest, and Delaware chapters of the AAPM; and the national AAPM were received. The major expense was the hiring of a legislative lobbyist, retired Senator Babe Schwartz. Once comments were received from reviewers, the

Practice Act was rewritten into a legislative template.

In 1989, the licensure bill, sponsored by Senator Chet Brooks and Representative Brad Wright, was submitted to the Texas legislature. Committee hearings were held and contacts were made per the lobbyist's expert guidance. The bill passed the legislature in 1989 but was not signed by then-Governor Bill Clements. Although eligible, it was not reopened during the 1989 special session called by the governor, who specified the agenda. In 1990, Anne Richards was elected governor of Texas, and the TMPS Practice Act was resubmitted to the 1991 legislature. The bill was passed by the legislature and signed by Governor Richards on May 28, 1991. The act created the Texas Board of Licensure for Professional Medical Physicists; the effective date was September 1, 1991. This landmark event established the first state requirement for medical physics licensure.

The Texas Board of Licensure for Professional Medical Physicists is administratively supported by the Texas Department of Health's Professional Licensing and Certification Division. The members of the Texas Licensure Board are appointed by the governor, and the first members, appointed by Governor Richards, were Stewart Bushong (chairman), Ann Wright (vice chairman), David Goff, Paul Murphy, and Wayne Wiatrowski (all medical physicists) and Ralph Blumhardt, Lester Peters, and Thomas Harle (all physicians).

At the first meeting of the Texas Board of Licensure in 1992, board members began developing rules for regulation of the practice of medical physics in Texas, for supervision of the application processing, and for development of a licensure examination. By August 1992, the initial rules were finalized. Rules are statements that interpret and implement provisions of a statute and define board procedures and the practice guidelines of the licensed profession.

5. Current requirements for Texas medical physicists licensure

Medical physicists residing anywhere in the United States are eligible to hold a Texas license, which qualifies them to practice medical physics in Texas. Texas offers licensure in four categories: diagnostic radiological physics, therapeutic radiological physics, medical nuclear physics, and medical health physics. Table 1 shows the distribution of Texas licenses as of 1995. At the time this table was developed, 449 medical physics licenses had been granted to Texas residents and 288 to residents of other states.

Originally, there were three ways to apply for a Texas medical physicist license: by the grandfather clause, by examination, or by reciprocity. The grandfather clause, which expired in September 1994, was adopted into legislation to ensure that anyone practicing medical physics at the time licensure became effective would be entitled to continue their practice with a license.

Table 1. Distribution of Texas Medical Physics Licenses as of 1995*

Licensure Category	Texas Resident		Out of State	
	Permanent License	Temporary License**	Permanent License	Temporary License
Diagnostic Radiological Physics	93	9	73	4
Therapeutic Radiological Physics	116	21	80	4
Medical Nuclear Physics	82	6	61	0
Medical Health Physics	115	7	66	0
Total	**406**	**43**	**280**	**8**

*Adapted from Bushong (1995).
**Medical physicists who do not qualify for permanent licensure may receive a temporary license, which is renewable annually for 3 years to allow the applicant to satisfy the requirements for permanent licensure.

The requirements for licensure by examination are: 1) a graduate degree in medical physics or in a Texas Board of Licensure-approved field, 2) 2 years full-time experience (within 5 years of the licensure application date) in the specialty category indicated on the application and 6 months additional full-time experience in each additional specialty category, 3) a passing score on the Texas Board of Licensure examination on state regulations and either national board certification in the specialty area(s) or a passing score on the Texas Board of Licensure examination in the specialty area(s), and 4) references from two physicists and one physician attesting to the applicant's professional ability.

The requirements for licensure by reciprocity are: 1) proof that the applicant is not a resident of Texas and is licensed in another state (Florida is the only other state with licensure at this time), 2) documentation of equivalent requirements as judged by the Texas Board of Licensure, and 3) references from two physicists and one physician attesting to the applicant's professional ability.

Individuals who do not have the experience to qualify for permanent licensure may apply for a temporary license. The temporary license may be renewed every year for 3 years. The requirements are: 1) a graduate degree in medical physics or in a Texas Board of Licensure-approved field, 2) references from two physicists and one physician attesting to the applicant's professional ability, and 3) sponsorship by a preceptor who is a fully licensed medical physicist and who will ensure that the temporary license holder acquires the necessary experience and who will take full responsibility for the temporary license holder's actions. Once the temporary license holder acquires the necessary experience, he or she may take the required examinations for permanent licensure.

More details on the procedures and requirements for receiving medical physicists licensure can be found at the Texas Department of Health Web site (www.tdh.state.tx.us/HCQS/PLC/physics.htm).

6. Credentialing in a profession

Whereas a license to practice in a profession is granted by a governmental body (typically the state legislature), a credential is granted by a local, private, supervisory board. A common example is the credentialing of a physician by a hospital board to practice a certain specialty or subset of a specialty on patients admitted to the institution. A license is required to practice in a licensed profession, but credentialing may or may not be required by one's institution. An individual must be licensed before he or she can be granted a credential, but the converse is not true. Credentialing of medical physicists is only required by a few institutions, usually only at larger institutions where several nonphysician staff have sought recognition for their professional expertise by the institution, thus achieving some protection through the bylaws of the institution.

The advantage of credentialing to the medical staff is that it establishes a due process of rules and laws that can be used to settle disputes that arise between the administration and the practitioner. In establishing credentialing, the governing board of the institution makes a commitment to nondiscriminatory practices in granting privileges to the practitioner. The practitioner's professional status is thus enhanced by becoming credentialed, and practice privileges are allowed as long as the practitioner adheres to the bylaws of the credentialing institution.

Credentialing requirements can vary significantly from one institution to another, so consistency in practice is not ensured. Credentialing is evaluated and granted by a committee composed of members of the institution's medical staff. To apply for a credential, the medical physicist must provide professional references from his or her previous employers, personal references, proof of specialty board certification and licensure (if applicable), proof of adequate health, and proof of medical insurability. As part of the application, the medical physicist requests privileges to practice medical physics. The format for that request can vary. It can be as broad as requesting permission to practice a specialty (e.g., diagnostic imaging physics) or as detailed as listing every service provided by the radiation therapy physicist.

7. Summary

Licensure and credentialing of medical physicists are processes still in development. Licensure of medical physicists is a state-government granted authorization that presently exists only in Texas and Florida. The benefits of licensure to the patient, public, and professional medical physicist dictate that we must continue to strive for adoption of medical physicist licensure by all states. In the interim, medical physicists can show their support for licensure by supporting national and state efforts, by becoming licensed in a license-issuing state until their state adopts licensure, and by supporting professional medical physicist associations.

Medical physicists should also actively participate in the credentialing process. If credentialing is not offered at your institution, it should be recommended through the medical staff office. As our profession matures, we can expect licensure and credentialing to be required of medical physicists as it is of physicians, dentists, and other health care providers.

References

American College of Medical Physics (1992) ACMP Resolution—Licensure for medical physicist. *American College of Medical Physics Newsletter* **Spring,** 6

Bushong S (1995) Report of Texas Board of Licensure for professional medical physicists. *American College of Medical Physics Newsletter* **Fall,** 5

Deye J (1985) Licensure of medical physicists. *Bulletin of the American College of Medical Physics* **2**(1),14-17

Mills M 1990 Editor's corner—Why licensure? *American College of Medical Physics Newsletter* **Spring,** 8

— (1991) Licensure Committee. *American College of Medical Physics Newsletter* **Spring,** 6

Wright A (1991) State licensure and the medical physicists. *American College of Medical Physics Newsletter* **Fall,** 7

Other resources

American College of Medical Physics (1989) Board of Chancellors Meeting. *Bulletin of the American College of Medical Physics* **1**(1),5-8

— (1992a) Letter to the Editor—Texas licensure. *American College of Medical Physics Newsletter* **Summer,** 4

— (1992b) Need for licensing as viewed from California. *American College of Medical Physics Newsletter* **Summer,** 4

— (1994) Update on licensure in Texas. *American College of Medical Physics Newsletter* **Winter,** 5

Landers R (1995) Florida licensure of medical radiological physicists. *American College of Medical Physics Newsletter* **Fall,** 4

Pipman Y (1994) Status of New York medical physics licensure effort. *American College of Medical Physics Newsletter* **Spring,** 7

David L. Goff, PhD

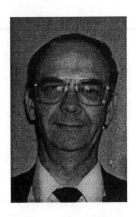

David L. Goff received his PhD in Engineering (Radiation Health) in 1969 from the University of Texas in Austin, TX. From 1968 to 1976, he worked as a clinical medical physicist and radiation safety officer for Santa Rosa Medical Center and Radiology Associates in San Antonio, TX, and from 1976 to 1979, he worked as a staff radiation physicist for Radiation Oncology of San Antonio. From 1979 to the present, Dr. Goff has served as President of Medical and Radiation Physics, Inc., a consulting firm serving central and south Texas. Dr. Goff has actively participated in professional activities. He is a Fellow of the ACMP and served as Chairman of its Board of Chancellors in 1992. He is also active in the AAPM and served as President of the Southwest Chapter in 1982. A well-respected professional medical physicist, Dr. Goff was appointed to serve on the inaugural Texas Board of Licensure for Professional Medical Physicists from 1992 to 1994.

Job Opportunities

Medical Physics Staffing for Diagnostic Imaging

Stewart C. Bushong, ScD

Department of Radiology, Baylor College of Medicine, Houston, TX

Abstract. The need for medical physics support for x-ray was not apparent until perhaps the 1960s. During the early years of the American Association of Physicists in Medicine, only a handful of that membership was engaged in the support of diagnostic imaging. With the introduction of ultrasound in the 1960s, computer tomography in the 1970s, magnetic resonance imaging in the 1980s, and the many advances in x-ray imaging during those three decades, medical physics support for diagnostic imaging became evermore evident and then essential. This report reviews the history of efforts to develop such medical physics support. The current practice and responsibilities of the diagnostic medical physicist are presented. Recommended medical physics staffing levels are reported from the practice protocols developed by the American Association of Physicists in Medicine, the American College of Medical Physics, and the American College of Radiology. The basic recommendation for staffing suggests that one diagnostic medical physicist is required for every 40 x-ray tubes.

1. Introduction

At the turn of the century, during the very early years of radiology, both diagnostic imaging and radiation therapy were carried out principally by scientists whom we would now identify as medical physicists. With the development of the physician practice of radiology, and in particular the practice of radiation oncology, the need for medical physics support was apparent. However, even radiation oncology did not come into its own until the 1950s with the introduction of cobalt teletherapy. Since that time, effective medical physics support for radiation oncology has been an undisputed requirement for the successful management of patients.

From the turn of the century until the 1960s, very little changed in the practice of diagnostic imaging, and what we recognize as medical physics support today was largely absent. However, the last several decades have witnessed an explosion of new imaging modalities employing evermore sophisticated technological apparatuses and methodology. Today, medical physics support for diagnostic imaging is also essential for the successful care of patients. Large health care facilities will require full-time on-site support. Community hospitals with limited medical imaging will require regularly scheduled consultative support. Most of this required medical physics support is technology driven, but the ever-increasing and complex radiation regulations also play a role.

2. A little history

Probably the first document to deal with medical physicists and their role in diagnostic imaging was a report published by the Hospital Physicists Association of the United Kingdom in 1973 entitled "Diagnostic x-ray protection: The role of the radiological protection advisor" (Hospital Physicists Association 1973). As the title stated, this document dealt primarily with protection from radiation rather than image quality. The report recommended that a medical physicist skilled in diagnostic imaging should be available to every hospital, at least on a consulting basis. That same year, the Joint Committee of the American College of Radiology (ACR) and the American Association of Physicists in Medicine (AAPM) on Manpower Needs in Medical Physics published a report entitled, "Status and future manpower needs of physicists in medicine in the United States" (Department of Health, Education and Welfare 1973). The committee was formed in 1969 for the purpose stated in the report title, and its work was based on a questionnaire mailed to the then 500 members of the AAPM. Figure 1, which is reproduced from that report, identifies the medical physics services required for x-ray imaging. Similar diagrams were developed for radiation therapy, nuclear medicine, and radiation safety.

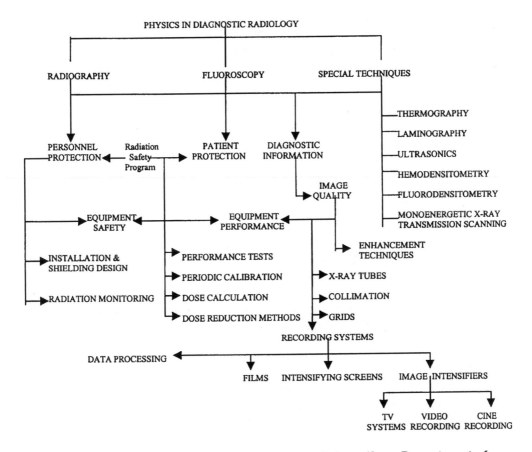

Figure 1. Medical physics services in diagnostic radiology (from Department of Health, Education and Welfare 1973).

At the time of this report, radiologists and medical physicists were practicing in all areas of radiology; specialization emerged in the late 1970s following the mandate to separate radiology residency programs into specialty areas, i.e., diagnostic radiology, nuclear medicine, and radiation oncology.

The six recommendations of the 1973 ACR-AAPM report were: 1) that at least one full-time medical physicist be provided for every 300 hospital beds; 2) that training should terminate in a master's or doctoral degree; 3) that the number of medical physicists should be doubled by 1983; 4) that medical physics training programs should be accredited; 5) that certification should be studied, particularly because of the diversity of fields in which medical physicists work; and 6) that courses in medical physics should be provided for other health care workers. These recommendations were largely met in subsequent years.

Both of these early reports struggled with terminology. The American Board of Radiology examination is for certification in radiological physics. The recommendation at that time was that physicists practice medical physics. There is a considerable difference between a radiological physicist and a medical physicist. Medical physicists have specialized training and knowledge that radiological physicists do not, and medical physics is a broader field of practice than radiological physics. The ACR-AAPM Committee offered the following description.

> "The term medical physics is not always interpreted consistently.
> Medical physics is defined as all applications of physics to any aspect of
> medicine. … medical physics includes the work physicists perform in the
> following well established areas of medicine: therapeutic radiology,
> diagnostic radiology, nuclear medicine, radiobiology, hospital health
> physics (radiation protection) and in the emerging fields of physiologic
> monitoring of patients, ultrasound, lasers, ophthalmology, thermography,
> information theory and biomedical engineering."

In the late 1970s, an ACR task group was formed to develop Current Procedural Terminology codes for diagnostic imaging medical physics. The four medical physicists and one radiologist who comprised the task group (Table 1) developed a number of codes, but the codes were never released for general use. Consequently, these codes never reached the American Medical Association approval phase and were never published as were successfully developed codes for radiation oncology, which are currently under attack.

Table 1. ACR Task Group for Development of Diagnostic Medical Physics Current Procedural Terminology Codes
Jack Krohmer, PhD, chairman Stewart Bushong, ScD George Callendine, PhD Norman Bailey, PhD Mark Mishkin, MD

In the early 1980s, William Hendee, PhD, a medical physicist, served as chairman of the Department of Radiology at the University of Colorado Medical School, Denver, CO. During his tenure, he developed and instituted a schedule of charges per procedure in order to fund diagnostic imaging medical physics on a systematic basis. Dr. Hendee's program was successful at the University of Colorado, but I am not aware of its adoption elsewhere.

3. The practice of diagnostic imaging medical physics

One of the first projects of the American College of Medical Physics (ACMP) after its formation by the AAPM in 1980 was formation of a task group to review staffing requirements and practice standards for imaging physics. The task group (Table 2) had three charges: 1) identify the practice activities of diagnostic medical physicists, 2) develop standards of practice for those areas, and 3) recommend appropriate staffing levels.

Table 2. ACMP Task Group for Development of Staffing Requirements and Practice Standards for Diagnostic Imaging Medical Physics

Stewart Bushong, ScD, chairman
Stephen Balter, PhD
Ted Fields, MS
Larry Rothenberg, PhD
Louis Wagner, PhD
      Consultants: John Domatti, MS
                    Sharon Glaze, MS
                    Joel Gray, PhD
                    Art Haus, MS

3.1. Practice activities of diagnostic imaging medical physicists

The practice of diagnostic medical physics can be identified either by type of service rendered, i.e., routine services (Table 3) or special/consulting services (Table 4) or by facility, i.e., research/teaching institutions, medical-center hospitals, or community hospitals.

Table 3. Routine Diagnostic Medical Physics Services
Radiographic performance monitoring Fluoroscopic performance monitoring Assessment of protective apparel Evaluation of personnel monitoring Regulatory compliance Patient protection and/or image quality control Computed tomography Magnetic resonance imaging Nuclear medicine imaging Mammography Diagnostic ultrasound Computed radiography

Table 4. Special/Consulting Diagnostic Imaging Medical Physics Services
Facility design
Purchase performance specifications
Acceptance testing
In-service training
Patient dose assessment

Special/consulting services are services that are provided on an as-needed basis. They are not routinely scheduled; rather, they are usually implemented in response to a special need. Table 4 includes a partial list of special/consulting services. An example of a special/consulting service is represented by an Internet notice posted in early 1997. A batch of lead contaminated with polonium had been shipped to manufacturers of protective lead aprons in 1995. Radiographers who wear these aprons can receive up to 6 mR/hr of radiation exposure at contact. It is not certain that these aprons have exposed personnel to excessive radiation; nevertheless, these aprons are on recall.

Another special/consulting service is facility design, an area that requires expert skill and competency such as is provided by the Baylor College of Medicine medical physics faculty in Houston, TX. The medical physicists at Baylor perform a considerable number of protective-barrier calculations for both single-room facilities and large medical-center hospitals. One of our faculty members, Ben Archer, PhD, is recognized as an expert in this area. Dose assessment is another important special/consulting service.

The mixture of routine and special/consulting services often depends on the type of facility involved. A research/teaching institution will have its own staff of diagnostic medical physicists performing, on average, more special consultation than is required in smaller health-care facilities. Most medical-center and community hospitals rely on private-practice diagnostic medical physicists for routine services, which are generally provided quarterly, semiannually, or annually. Special/consultative services tend to be required less often.

3.2. Standards of practice for diagnostic medical physicists

The ACMP task group met its second charge by stimulating the publication of several diagnostic medical physics practice protocols (Table 5). These publications somewhat mirror the Standards of Practice documents developed by the ACR for the practice of radiology. Although some of the ACR standards mention the requirement for medical physics, they are not very proscriptive.

At the time the ACMP practice protocols appeared, the AAPM was busy publishing a number of documents (see Table 6 for a partial list) to assist the diagnostic medical physicist with the technical aspects of implementing the suggested practice protocols. All of the documents listed in Tables 5 and 6 are required references for the practice of diagnostic medical physics.

Table 5. Practice Protocols of the ACMP

Radiation Control and Quality Assurance Surveys: Diagnostic Radiology—A Suggested Protocol
ACMP Report No. 1; January 1986

Radiation Control and Quality Assurance Surveys: Magnetic Resonance Imaging—A Suggested Protocol
ACMP Report No. 5; June 1989

Radiation Control and Quality Assurance Surveys: Mammography—A Suggested Protocol
ACMP Report No. 4; February 1989

Radiation Control and Quality Assurance Surveys: Medical Laser Systems
ACMP Report No. 6; October 1990

Radiation Control and Quality Assurance Surveys: Nuclear Medicine—A Suggested Protocol
ACMP Report No. 3; January 1986

Table 6. Practice Protocols of the AAPM

Basic Quality Control in Diagnostic Radiology
AAPM Report No. 4; November 1977

Pulse Echo Ultrasound Imaging Systems: Performance Tests and Criteria
AAPM Report No. 9; November 1980

A Standard Format for Digital Image Exchange
AAPM Report No. 10; March 1982

Evaluation of Radiation Exposure Levels in Cine Cardiac Catheterization Laboratories
AAPM Report No. 12; January 1984

Performance Evaluation and Quality Assurance in Digital Subtraction Angiography
AAPM Report No. 15; May 1985

Site Planning for Magnetic Resonance Imaging Systems
AAPM Report No. 20; December 1986

Rotating Scintillation Camera Spect Acceptance Testing and Quality Control
AAPM Report No. 22; June 1987

Protocols for the Radiation Safety Surveys of Diagnostic Radiological Equipment
AAPM Report No. 25; May 1988

Quality Assurance Methods and Phantoms for Magnetic Resonance Imaging
AAPM Report No. 28; May 1990

Equipment Requirements and Quality Control for Mammography
AAPM Report No. 29; August 1990

Standardized Methods for Measuring Diagnostic X-ray Exposures
AAPM Report No. 31; July 1990

Table 6. Practice Protocols of the AAPM (continued)
Staffing Levels and Responsibilities of Physicists in Diagnostic Radiology AAPM Report No. 33; April 1991 Acceptance Testing of Magnetic Resonance Imaging Systems AAPM Report No. 34; March 1992 Recommendations on Performance Characteristics of Diagnostic Exposures Meters AAPM Report No. 35; March 1992 Specification and Acceptance Testing of Computed Tomography Scanners AAPM Report No. 39; May 1993 The Role of the Clinical Medical Physicist in Diagnostic Radiology AAPM Report No. 42; January 1994

3.3. Diagnostic medical physics staffing

The ACMP task group made only a modest beginning in its charge to identify appropriate staffing levels. The task group could not arrive at a consensus, and therefore, the assignment was transferred to a new joint ACMP-AAPM committee. The new committee was directed to collect contemporary data on existing staffing levels and use that as a basis for new recommendations (Table 7).

Table 7. Joint ACMP-AAPM Task Group for Recommendations on Diagnostic Medical Physics Staffing

Edward Nickoloff, ScD, chairman
Stewart Bushong, ScD
Charles Kelsey, PhD
James Keriakes, PhD
Mark Mishkin, MD
Larry Rothenberg, PhD
Louis Wagner, PhD
        Consultants: James Deye, PhD
                      Thomas Payne, PhD
                      Raymond Tanner, PhD

The business of putting numbers to staffing was given considerable status with publication of the "Blue Book" (Inter-Society Council for Radiation Oncology 1991), a report that dealt with staffing in radiation oncology. This committee report was sponsored by a number of physician organizations and the AAPM. A particularly effective recommendation in the report was that one medical physicist should be available for every 400 patients. This ratio, 1:400, has become a rather widely accepted value.

The joint ACMP-AAPM task group tried, in some fashion, to mimic what the radiation oncology task group had done in the past. Over a 3-year period, a considerable amount of data was collected in an attempt to determine how many diagnostic medical physicists were required to provide routine and special/consulting services that would comply with practice standards. The result was a report entitled,

"Recommendations on physics staffing for diagnostic radiology" (American Institute of Physics 1993). The resulting recommendations identified the number of x-ray tubes per physicist rather than the number of patients per physicist.

An exceptional amount of practice data were generated from this report, and although the staffing criteria are based on x-ray tubes per physicist, all diagnostic medical physics services are included. It was felt that the number of x-ray tubes used per physicist was a reasonably common indicator of not only x-ray imaging staffing requirements but staffing requirements in other areas as well, such as, magnetic resonance imaging, diagnostic ultrasound imaging, and nuclear medicine. The report also recognizes that use of a radiographic x-ray tube will require less support by a diagnostic medical physicist than will computed tomography, computed radiography, or digital fluoroscopy.

The staffing level recommended in the American Institute of Physics Report is one diagnostic medical physicist for every 40 x-ray tubes. In addition to accounting for different types of x-ray tubes, as previously described, this recommendation is intended to satisfy all routine and special/consulting services involved in diagnostic medical physics practice. However, the report does recognize that this recommended staffing level may vary according to facility size; and thus, modification is left to the judgement of the professional and administrative staff. For example, a research/teaching institution may require a ratio of 1:30 (physicist:x-ray tubes) or even 1:20, depending on the respective research or educational goals. On the other hand, a community hospital may require a diagnostic medical physicist only twice a year for a ratio of 1:60 or as low as 1:100. For facilities with heavy diagnostic ultrasound or nuclear medicine practices, recommended staffing levels are 1 physicist to 50 ultrasound imagers and 1 physicist to 8 gamma cameras. The nomogram shown in Figure 2 can be used to determine diagnostic imaging medical physics staffing levels. An example is given for a representative hospital having 38 x-ray tubes, 4 diagnostic ultrasound imagers, and 3 gamma cameras.

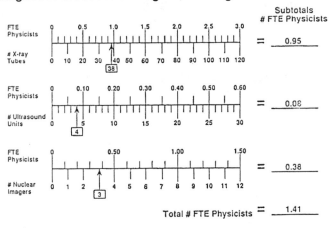

Figure 2. Worksheet to determine recommended physics staffing for diagnostic radiology. FTE, full-time equivalent.

The ACMP-AAPM report was published before the Mammography Quality Standards Act was introduced. Although no published data are available regarding the diagnostic medical physicist and the Mammography Quality Standards Act, each mammography imager requires approximately 2 days attention by a medical physicist per year.

4. Conclusion

How realistic are the American Institute of Physics staffing level recommendations? Our experience at Baylor is that most hospitals are very understaffed. With changes in the delivery of health care and the increasing complexity of regulations, more hospitals are outsourcing their diagnostic medical physics services. The result is less cost; but the question is, "Are the services within practice guidelines?" Currently at Baylor, 5 diagnostic medical physicists provide special/consulting services to approximately 250 health care facilities of various sizes. The total x-ray tube count is approximately 1200, resulting in a 1:240 ratio.

At Ben Taub General Hospital, Houston, TX, the principal teaching institution for Baylor, there are 80 x-ray tubes, 8 diagnostic ultrasound imagers, 1 magnetic resonance imager, and 4 gamma cameras. A nomogram calculation of these values suggests the need for 2.65 full-time equivalent (FTE) diagnostic imaging medical physicists. The available staff is 1.5 or a ratio of 1:53 x-ray tubes.

At The Methodist Hospital, Houston, TX, another one of Baylor's teaching institutions, there are 130 x-ray tubes, 9 diagnostic ultrasound imagers, 4 magnetic resonance imagers, and 8 gamma cameras. There are 2.5 FTE diagnostic imaging medical physicists at this institution. A nomogram calculation of these values results in a recommendation for 4.45 FTE diagnostic medical physicists.

Clearly, more data and more effort are required to formalize the diagnostic medical physicist staffing requirement recommendations.

REFERENCES

American Institute of Physics (1993) "Recommendations on physics staffing for diagnostic radiology," A report of the Trilateral Committee of the AAPM, ACMP, and ACR Commission on Physics. Woodbury, NY:AIP

Department of Health, Education and Welfare (1973) "Status and future manpower need of physicists in medicine in the United States," DHEW Publication No. FDA 73-8014

Hospital Physicists Association (1973) "Diagnostic x-ray protection: The role of the Radiological Protection Advisor," HPA Report No. 9. Bristol, UK: HPA

Inter-Society Council for Radiation Oncology (1991) "Radiation oncology in integrated cancer management." Philadelphia, PA:ACR

Stewart C. Bushong, ScD

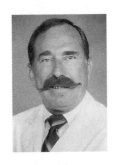

Stewart C. Bushong received his ScD in Radiation Health from the University of Pittsburgh. Dr. Bushong is presently Professor and Chief, Section of Radiological Science, Department of Radiology at Baylor College of Medicine. Dr. Bushong is a Fellow of the ACMP, the AAPM, and the ACR. He has made significant contributions to professional medical physics through service exemplified by having served on the Board of Directors of the American Board of Medical Physics, AAPM, and the Health Physics Society; as Chairman of the ACMP; and as Chairman of the Texas Board of Licensure for Professional Medical Physicists. Dr. Bushong is active locally, nationally, and internationally as a consultant in radiological physics. He is known as an educator and is particularly well known in the fields of diagnostic imaging and radiation protection, areas in which he has published 140 scientific papers and 23 books.

Medical Physics Staffing Requirements for Radiation Oncology Physics Services

Richard G. Lane, PhD

Department of Radiation Physics, The University of Texas M. D. Anderson Cancer Center, Houston, TX

Abstract. Over the past several years, an increase in the number of facilities, the number of treatment machines, and the complexity of treatment techniques in both external-beam treatments and in brachytherapy has resulted in an increase in the number of medical physicists employed in radiation oncology. Organizations representing medical physicists have attempted to keep up with this growth by publishing reports on the scientific and professional aspects of medical physics in radiation oncology. Some of the documents published by these organizations are clearly standards, whereas others are published as recommendations. The overall goal of these publications is to provide performance standards for clinical medical physics activities in radiation oncology. The recommendations regarding patient care activities provide information that can be used to determine medical physics staffing levels.

1. Introduction

Over the past several years, the field of radiation oncology has undergone tremendous growth. An increase in the number of facilities and in the number of treatment machines has been accompanied by an increasing complexity of treatment techniques in both external-beam treatments and in brachytherapy. Because of this growth, increasing numbers of medical physicists have been employed in radiation oncology.

Organizations representing medical physicists have attempted to keep up with this growth by publishing reports on the scientific and professional aspects of medical physics in radiation oncology. For example, in 1993 the American Association of Physicists in Medicine (AAPM) published a report entitled "The role of a physicist in radiation oncology" (American Association of Physicists in Medicine 1993), which expands on a report published in 1986 entitled "The roles, responsibilities, and status of the clinical medical physicist" (American Association of Physicists in Medicine 1986). These are only two in a long series of AAPM reports on the practice of medical physics in general and on radiation oncology physics in particular.

The AAPM reports that make specific recommendations regarding the scientific aspects of radiation oncology physics are usually published in *Medical Physics* to ensure the widest possible dissemination of information throughout the medical physics community. Examples include, Reports of AAPM Radiation Therapy Committee (RTC) Task Group Nos. 21 and 25 (American Association of Physicists in Medicine 1983, 1991), which presented recommendations on the calibration of photon and electron beams and the clinical application of electron beams, respectively. More recently, Reports of AAPM RTC Task Group No. 45, "Code of practice for radiotherapy accelerators," and Task Group No. 40, "Comprehensive QA for radiation oncology," (American Association of Physicists in Medicine 1994a, 1994b) provided extensive recommendations on these critically important radiation oncology physics activities.

Other organizations publishing reports, recommendations, and standards on radiation oncology include:

- American College of Medical Physics (ACMP) (1986,1987)
- American College of Radiology (ACR) (1990)
- Hospital Physicists Association (1969)
- International Atomic Energy Agency (1970)
- International Commission on Radiation Protection (1985)
- International Commission on Radiation Units and Measurements (1985)
- International Electrotechnical Commission (1989)
- Nordic Association of Clinical Physicists (1980)
- National Council of Radiation Protection and Measurements (1981)

Some of the documents published by these organizations are clearly standards, whereas others are published as recommendations or reports. The overall goal of these publications is to provide performance standards for clinical medical physics activities in radiation oncology. They are required reading for the practicing radiation oncology physicist.

By making recommendations regarding patient care activities and the minimum criteria to be met in performing these activities, these publications also provide information that can be used to determine medical physics staffing levels.

This chapter reviews current documents that can help the practicing medical physicist evaluate staffing based on patient load, standards of practice, and the recommendations of American and European medical physics organizations.

2. Historical staffing levels

In 1997, the ACR, as part of its Patterns of Care Study, published the eighth in a series of surveys on the structure of radiation oncology, which included a census of facilities in the United States at which megavoltage radiotherapy is delivered (Owen et al. 1997). These surveys include information on facilities, treatment machines, personnel, patient load, facility capabilities, and trends over time. Although the surveys include information dating back to 1974, medical physics staffing data were first included in 1983. Using the most recent survey, we can determine historical trends in medical physics staffing levels up to the year 1994, the last year for which data are available.

Table 1 shows the status of radiation oncology in the United States in 1994. It includes the number of facilities, treatment machines, radiation oncologists, physicists, dosimetrists, and radiation therapists available to treat patients in hospitals or freestanding centers. The last column (multi-unit) lists the number of these resources at facilities that had more than one treatment unit. Note that in 1994, there was approximately one physicist per facility and that each physicist was responsible for the work associated with approximately two accelerators.

Table 1. Structure of Radiation Oncology in 1994

	Total	Hospital	Free-standing	Multi-unit
Facilities	1542	1047	462	851
Linear accelerators	2425	2031	650	2056
Cobalt units	314	251	54	248
Radiation oncologists	2777	2091	613	1934
Physicists (FTE)	1349	1129	180	1114
Dosimetrists	1314	1013	271	1004
Radiation therapists	7167	5538	1478	5371

FTE, full-time equivalent

Trends in the numbers of radiation oncology facilities, equipment, and staff from 1983 to 1994 are shown in Table 2. Also included are the number of patients treated and the percent increase in numbers of patients, facilities, equipment, and staff over this time period. Note that the numbers of radiation oncology facilities, equipment, and staff increased at a greater rate than did the number of patients treated. For example, the numbers of medical physicists increased 1.5 times that of the increase in patient load, and the number of dosimetrists increased 5 times that of the increase in patient load. By 1994, the number of patients treated per staff member was 202 patients per radiation oncologist, 415 patients per medical physicist, 426 patients per dosimetrist, and 78 patients per therapist.

Table 2. Trends in Radiation Oncology

Trends	1983	1986	1990	1994	% change '83-'94
New patients	400K	444K	492K	560K	40.0
Facilities	1083	1144	1321	1542	42.4
Treatment machines	1762	1965	2397	2744	55.7
Radiation oncologists	1904	2055	2335	2777	45.9
Physicists (FTE)	842	935	1092	1349	60.2
Dosimetrists	438	523	1078	1314	200.0
Therapists	3648	4242	5353	7167	96.5

FTE, full-time equivalent

3. Staffing-level recommendations

Table 3 shows the recommended staffing levels for radiation oncology as published in the December 1991 report "Radiation oncology in integrated cancer management" called the "Blue Book" (Inter-Society Council for Radiation Oncology 1991). This report was sponsored by the AAPM, ACMP, ACR, and other medical societies involved with the practice of radiation oncology. Not unexpectedly, the staffing levels recommended by this group of associations were consistent with levels prevalent at the time. These recommended staffing levels exclude all teaching, research, and clinical development efforts usually found in academic facilities. In addition, there is no mention of special radiation oncology procedures, which are becoming an integral part of modern radiation oncology practice and which require extensive medical physics involvement.

Table 3. Blue Book Staffing Recommendations: Personnel
Requirements for Clinical Radiation Oncology

Category	Staffing Level
Radiation oncologists	One per 200-250 patients treated annually
Medical physicist	One per 400 patients treated annually
Dosimetrist	One per 300 patients treated annually
Therapist	Two for up to 25 patients treated daily/machine (approximately one per 125 patients treated annually)
Brachytherapy technician	As needed
Treatment aid technician	As needed
Engineer	One per two-megavoltage machines

Recently, a joint working group from the European Society for Therapeutic Radiology and Oncology and the European Federation of Organizations for Medical Physics assessed the medical physics staffing levels necessary to support radiation oncology (European Society for Therapeutic Radiology and Oncology/European Federation of Organizations for Medical Physics 1996). Their recommendations are summarized in Table 4. This report separates the physics effort required for quality assurance of major equipment from that required in support of patient treatment. In addition, the report affirms the supervisory role of the radiation oncology physicist by emphasizing that a qualified medical physicist must make up approximately half the total physics staff effort needed for any particular medical physics activity.

Table 5 provides examples of staffing levels for three different size facilities. Note that the recommended staffing levels differ from those of the Blue Book recommendations (Table 3) principally because the latter does not include the physics quality assurance duties associated with brachytherapy equipment and planning systems as well as the brachytherapy patient procedures themselves. As is true of the Blue Book recommendations, these staffing-level recommendations do not include any teaching or development efforts.

Table 4. European Society for Therapeutic Radiology and Oncology/European Federation of Organizations for Medical Physics Staffing Recommendations*

Subject	Total Staff (FTE)	Minimum Number QMP (FTE)
Accelerator	0.88	0.37
Cobalt unit	0.34	0.14
Kilovoltage	0.07	0.03
Afterloader	0.42	0.18
Treatment planning		
Teletherapy	0.38	0.16
Brachytherapy	0.08	0.04
100 patients per year		
Teletherapy	0.27	0.11
Brachytherapy	0.22	0.09

*Recommended minimum medical physics staffing levels for routine clinical activities in radiation oncology. QMP, qualified medical physicist; FTE, full-time equivalent.

Table 5. Examples of Recommended Staffing Levels*

Institution	Single Unit	Modest Hospital	Large Hospital
Equipment	1 accelerator	2 accelerators	4 accelerators
	1 simulator	1 afterloader	2 afterloaders
	1 RTP	1 simulator	1 simulator
		1 RTP	1 CT-simulator
			3 RTP
Patients per year	350	600	1200 radiotherapy
		50	200 brachytherapy
Staffing			
Qualified medical physicist	1.0	1.92	4.08
Total staff	2.5	4.59	9.78

*Calculation of typical staffing levels. RTP, radiotherapy planning system.

4. Work values for radiation oncology physics services

Because of the direct patient care responsibilities of the radiation oncology physicist, the American Medical Association (AMA) has included billing codes for medical physics procedures in its Current Procedural Terminology manual (American Medical Association 1997). This manual lists activities performed by the medical physicist when caring for the patient and the billing codes used for those activities.

These codes were developed to aid in the compensation of physicians in all specialties, but they also address technical activities done in support of the professional medical procedure. Most medical physics codes include a professional component that applies to physician's fees and a technical component that applies to the fees hospitals charge for work done by the physicist and dosimetrist as well as the use of equipment required to perform that work. It is essential to understand that only AMA-coded activities will be reimbursed by any third-party payer (Medicare and insurance companies). All radiation oncology physics activities, including testing, commissioning, and quality assurance measurements done in support of the actual clinical activity, must be represented by one of these codes. Table 6 lists the AMA Current Procedural Terminology codes for all clinical medical physics activities in radiation oncology.

In 1995, the AAPM and the ACMP contracted with Abt Associates (Cambridge, MA), to study the time and effort required of medical physicists to perform the activities listed in Table 6. The results were published under the title "The Abt study of medical physicists work values for radiation oncology physics services" (Abt Associates Inc. 1995). A thorough review of this extensive document is beyond the scope of this paper, but I strongly recommend that radiation oncology physicists read and understand both the description of the study process and the study results. Table 7 extracts from the Abt study some of the data listing the time required, both non-procedural and procedural, to perform selected AMA-coded medical physics services in radiation oncology. Non-procedural time is the time involved in obtaining data and maintaining quality assurance standards. Procedural time is that time actually required to perform the procedure. Because of the way the study was structured, the total time does not necessarily represent the sum of the procedural and the non-procedural time. Using these data for all the medical physics codes, the required staffing level for any radiation oncology physics program can be determined from the number of coded procedures performed annually and the time required to perform the procedure.

5. Radiation oncology special procedures

None of the staffing level recommendations described above, including those developed through the Abt study, address the vast majority of radiation oncology special procedures, which are increasingly coming into use. High-dose-rate remote afterloading brachytherapy, total-skin irradiation, total-body irradiation, three-dimensional conformal radiation treatment planning, stereotactic radiosurgery, intraopertive radiation therapy, and stereotactic brachytherapy all require extensive medical physics involvement. The medical physics resources required to perform these procedures and to support patient treatment have been surveyed by the ACMP, and the results of the survey have been published as an ACMP task group report entitled, "Survey of physics resources for radiation oncology special procedures" (American College of Medical Physics 1998).

Table 6. American Medical Association Current Procedural Terminology Codes for Medical Radiation Physics, Dosimetry, Treatment Devices, and Special Services

Procedure	CPT Code
Basic radiation dosimetry calculation	77300
Teletherapy isodose plan:	
Simple	77305
Intermediate	77310
Complex	77315
Brachytherapy isodose calculation:	
Simple	77326
Intermediate	77327
Complex	77328
Treatment devices:	
Simple	77332
Intermediate	77333
Complex	77334
Special teletherapy port	77321
Special dosimetry	77331
Continuing medical radiation physics consultation	77336
Special medical radiation physics consultation	77370

CPT, Current Procedural Terminology

Table 7. Results of the Abt Study of Medical Physicist Work Values for Radiation Oncology Physics Services*

Code	Procedure	Non-Procedural	Procedural	Total
77300	Basic calculation	0.38	0.17	0.63
77315	Complex plan	0.38	0.50	1.15
77327	Complex brachytherapy plan	0.83	3.00	3.87
77334	Complex treatment device	0.04	0.25	0.34
77336	Continuing consultation	N/A	1.50	1.50
77370	Special consultation	N/A	4.00	4.00

*Median time in hours to perform medical physics services.

6. Summary

There is extensive literature available to assist the medical physicist in both the scientific and the professional aspects of radiation oncology physics. Using this essential information, the radiation oncology physicist can decide what policies and procedures are required to perform the medical physics activities necessary to ensure quality patient care and patient safety in radiation oncology. Based on these decisions, the medical physicist can determine the required staffing level.

It is critical that adequate medical physics staffing levels are in place to meet the needs of the department. Published staffing-level recommendations, workload studies, and manpower surveys all help to justify radiation oncology physics resources to meet the requirements of each situation. However, it is important to remember that these recommendations result from surveys conducted by interested parties. Others involved in staffing decisions also have surveys available to them. Department chairmen, department administrators, and hospital administrators all have access to formal or informal surveys of departmental characteristics, including medical physics staffing. The radiation oncology physicist must argue the need for adequate staffing by demonstrating the actual time involved in the work required and the consequences of inadequate staffing.

References

Abt Associates Inc. (1995) "The Abt study of medical physicists work values for radiation oncology physics services." Cambridge, MA:Abt Associates Inc.

American Association of Physicists in Medicine (1983) "A protocol for the determination of absorbed dose from high energy photon and electron beams," Report of AAPM Radiation Therapy Committee Task Group No. 21. *Medical Physics* **10**,741-771

— (1986) "The roles, responsibilities, and status of the clinical medical physicist," AAPM Report. New York, NY:AIP

— (1991) "Clinical electron-beam dosimetry," Report of AAPM Radiation Therapy Committee Task Group No. 25, AAPM Report No. 32. *Medical Physics* **18**,73-109

— (1993) "The role of a physicist in radiation oncology," AAPM Report No. 38. New York, NY:AIP

— (1994a) "Code of practice for radiotherapy accelerators," Report of AAPM Radiation Therapy Task Group No. 45. *Medical Physics* **21**,1093-1122

— (1994b) "Comprehensive QA for radiation oncology," Report of AAPM Radiation Therapy Task Group No. 40. *Medical Physics* **21**,581-618

American College of Medical Physics (1986) "Radiation control and quality assurance in radiation oncology: A suggested protocol," ACMP Report No. 2. Reston, VA:ACMP
— (1998) "Survey of physics resources for radiation oncology special procedures," ACMP Task Group Report. Reston, VA:ACMP

American College of Radiology (1990) "Standards for radiation oncology." Philadelphia, PA:ACR

American Medical Association (1997) Current Procedural Terminology. Chicago, IL:AMA

European Society for Therapeutic Radiology and Oncology/European Federation of Organizations for Medical Physics (1996) "Quality assurance in radiotherapy: The importance of medical physics staffing levels," ESTRO/EFOMP Joint Task Group Recommendation. *Radiotherapy and Oncology* **41**,89-94

Hospital Physics Association (1969) A code of practice for the dosimetry of 2-35 MV x-rays and Cs-137 and Co-60 gamma ray beams. *Physics in Medicine and Biology* **14**,1-8

International Atomic Energy Agency (1970) "Manual of dosimetry in radiotherapy," IAEA Report No. 110. Vienna, Austria:IAEA

International Commission on Radiation Protection (1985) "Protection of patients in radiotherapy," ICRP Report No. 24. Washington DC:ICRP

International Commission on Radiation Units and Measurements (1985) "Dose volume specification for reporting intracavitary therapy in gynecology," ICRU Report No. 38. Bethesda, MD:ICRU

International Electrotechnical Commission (1989) "Medical electron accelerators— Functional performance characteristics," IEC Publication 976. Geneva, Switzerland:IEC

Inter-Society Council for Radiation Oncology (1991) "Radiation oncology in integrated cancer management." Philadelphia, PA:ACR

National Council on Radiation Protection and Measurements (1981) "Dosimetry of x-ray and gamma ray beams for radiation therapy in the energy range 10 keV to 50 MeV," NCRP Report No. 69. Washington DC:NCRP

Nordic Association of Clinical Physicists (1980) Procedures in external beam radiation therapy: Dosimetry with electron and photon beams with maximum energy between 1 and 50 MeV. *Acta Radiologica Oncology* **19,**55-79

Owen JB, Coia LR, and Hanks GE (1997) Structure of radiation oncology in the United States in 1994. *International Journal of Radiation Oncology, Biology, Physics* **39**,179-185

Richard G. Lane, PhD

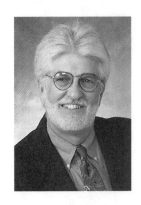

Richard G. Lane received his PhD in Medical Physics from the University of California at Los Angeles in 1970. He then joined the faculty of the University of Wisconsin as an Assistant Professor in the Department of Medical Physics. In 1975, he went to the University of New Mexico where he attained the rank of Professor in the Department of Radiology and served as Head of Radiotherapy Physics in the Cancer Research and Treatment Center from 1978 to 1985. From 1985 to 1998, Dr. Lane was a Professor in the Department of Radiation Oncology and Director of the Division of Physics and Engineering at the University of Texas Medical Branch in Galveston, TX. In 1998, Dr. Lane became Group Leader of External Beam Therapy Services at The University of Texas M. D. Anderson Cancer Center in Houston, TX. Dr. Lane has published over 60 scientific articles, book chapters, and conference proceedings. He is a Fellow of the AAPM, having served on its Board of Directors, as a member of several committees, and as president of two local chapters. Dr. Lane also is active in the ACMP and ACR Commission on Medical Physics. He is presently chair of the Commission on Accreditation of Medical Physics Education Programs, Inc. Residency Education Program Review Committee. He is highly regarded for his expertise in clinical radiation oncology physics.

The Job Search and Marketing Yourself*

Barbara Walters, BSc

Management Recruiters International Inc., Oklahoma City, OK

Abstract. A job search should never be a random activity consigned to luck and happenstance. Instead, the search needs to be a well thought out plan conducted by an individual who has a firm grasp of the nature of his or her personal strengths and weaknesses.

1. Introduction

This article summarizes the job search process and emphasizes some key points that I consider particularly important. There are as many viewpoints on this subject as there are people who have ever accepted a job. What I offer in this article are observations based on 20 years of successful recruiting experience. It is impossible to cover every contingency or situation you might encounter. In fact, I may not cover the topics you consider essential, but I will cover the most salient points.

2. What makes you marketable?

2.1. Education

A master's degree in medical physics from a program accredited by the Commission on Accreditation of Medical Physics Education Programs, Inc. (CAMPEP) is a must for a lucrative career. In some instances, a PhD degree is essential, but that is an individual career choice.

In the best of all possible worlds, your education will be accompanied by some very basic training. It has never ceased to amaze me that some medical physicists graduate from a medical physics program and cannot even perform morning quality assurance on a linear accelerator. Before beginning your job search, it is imperative that you evaluate your skill level. You should know some basic dosimetry and how to independently calibrate a linear accelerator. If you lack sufficient experience in these areas, it would be prudent to enroll in a residency program so you can learn these skills. If you decide to seek employment without the benefit of continued training, you have a responsibility to make sure that you are fully qualified for any position you accept. It is unfortunate, but many of the people making hiring decisions do not have the vaguest idea what medical physicists do or of the importance of their competency. Ultimately, you will be the one who will determine if you are sufficiently experienced to perform a job safely and competently.

---

* The opinions presented here are not necessarily endorsed by Management Recruiters International Inc.

2.2. Attitude

Some will say that you should not appear too eager on an interview. Hogwash! Enthusiasm is one of the most marketable attributes an applicant can possess. This is true at any stage of your career, but it is essential for new graduates. Your attitude must imply that you really want the job. A laid-back "you'll be lucky if you manage to hire me" demeanor will not serve your purpose. Also, never pretend to be someone you are not or to know something that you do not know. You can best influence the decision-making process by projecting an enthusiastic, honest, sincere attitude. You can always turn down an offer you do not want, but you cannot retrieve an offer that has been lost because you projected the wrong attitude.

2.3. Personal presentation

You will have three opportunities to make a first impression: with your resumé, your first telephone conversation, and when you present yourself for the face-to-face interview.

Your resumé does not have to be fancy, but it should be concise and well written and typed in a font that is easy to read (not too small, not too elaborate). The resumé should stress your accomplishments rather than your duties. Additional details about the resumé are found in Section 4, "Conquering the resumé."

Your first telephone interview can be difficult and intimidating. You are selling yourself, and if you have studied the product, you should do well. Aim to be personable and confident. Remember that language becomes a major factor when you are speaking to an interviewer by telephone. If the interviewer cannot understand you, he will assume that patients also will be unable to understand you. Practice is essential, and some speaking-skills training may be necessary. Talk "to" the interviewer, not "at" him or her. When you are interviewing by telephone, stand in front of a mirror, and talk to the person you see. This will create for you the feeling of having a conversation with "someone" rather than just a voice and will allow you to monitor yourself. Are you smiling or frowning? The interviewer will be able to hear this in your tone. Are you talking too much, interrupting the interviewer? Think about the things you are likely to do wrong and write yourself notes. Post the notes on the mirror to remind yourself to check for these behaviors.

Evaluate your appearance prior to the on-site interview. A conservative look is best. Hair should be neatly trimmed and styled. Men should make sure that any facial hair also is neatly trimmed and not excessive. Your attire should be well fitting and attractive, but not flashy. A suit (for men and women) is most appropriate, but in some instances, a navy blue sport coat, white shirt, and gray or tan slacks for men or a business-style, dark-toned dress for women is acceptable. Personal hygiene is also important. The goal is to project a clean, tidy look. Beware of personal preferences that might offend. I represented a person years ago who did not get a job because her potential employer was allergic to her perfume. She made him sneeze! If you are an expresso addict, make sure that your breath does not reek of coffee. One of my candidates unsuccessfully searched for a job for months in the nuclear medicine field. He was overweight and tended to arrive at interviews soaked in nervous perspiration. He also was negligent about basic hygiene. Although his credentials were impeccable, interviewers found him offensive.

Years ago, I interviewed the girl with the black nail polish, the man wearing the peacock blue cowboy boots and a pen stripe suit, and the woman with enough jewelry to make Tiffany's jealous. In fact, I had to find a place to hang her mink coat. I do not remember much else about these people or their skills. They will remain eternally as symbols of interviewing disasters. In general, make sure you will not be remembered for any reason other than your skills and personality. Be sure you are totally free of any personal characteristics that could be annoying or distracting. A sincere, nonbiased friend, colleague, or family member can be a valuable resource in helping you evaluate your appearance.

2.4. Communication skills

One cannot overestimate the importance of effective communication. Some people expect physicists to be odd looking, like the "nutty professor" who wears a stained lab coat complete with a pocket protector filled with pens and measuring devices. They may assume a physicist has limited social skills and conversational ability. Imagine their surprise when you, the modern, informed physicist, arrives at their facility. You are well-spoken, well-dressed, and well-groomed, and you have amicable interpersonal skills.

Learn the language of the country where you wish to work. Your language skills will impact your ability to get the job and salary you want. No amount of legislation will keep people from deciding against hiring you if they cannot understand you! Increasingly, radiation therapy physicists are being asked to visit with patients during the treatment process. People tend to be poor listeners to begin with, and when they are worried or feeling ill, the ability to listen suffers further. You must become fluent in the local language!

3. Preparing for the job search

3.1. Self evaluation

The more decisions you make before you actually begin interviewing the easier it will be to find and accept the right position. This process best begins with self evaluation. Initiate a discovery process. Assess your personal strengths and weaknesses. Ask friends, family members, instructors, and your significant other to help you in this process. It is an oddity of human nature that criticisms are more easily internalized than praise. Allow yourself to acknowledge your good points, and be willing to analyze the bad points. This introspective approach will enable you to formulate your own feature/benefit profile. There are three ground rules to remember when developing a feature/benefit profile.

- Rule 1: A feature is a fact about you that you can use to position yourself as a unique resource. A feature might be your degree, an accomplishment, a special skill or talent, your good looks, your wonderful voice, or your exceptional aptitude for math.

- Rule 2: A benefit is a value-added result for the organization based on one of your features.

- Rule 3: Any one feature may produce one or more benefits.

Developing a feature/benefit profile can be a frustrating experience. When you have diligently worked on it and feel like junking the entire project, throw the paperwork into a drawer; work on it again when you have regained your composure and a more optimistic attitude. When you complete your profile, internalize it; believe it. Use it to start speaking about yourself in a more confident, matter-of-fact manner.

Once your strengths have become part of your spoken vocabulary, consider your other distinguishing characteristics. Each of us is different, and what works best for me will not necessarily work for everyone. For, example, if you work best in quiet environments where you are free to think and work at your own pace, you probably will not fare well in a mega clinic performing 120 external-beam treatments per day staffed by only two medical physicists and one medical dosimetrist. Conversely, you might be recognized as one of the best in your field should you work in a less hectic atmosphere. These aspects of your personality are neither good nor bad but need to be recognized when deciding which employment situations to pursue.

When tallying up your balance sheet, acknowledge those parts of your character or skill set that need to be improved. Start working on a conscious plan to achieve improvement in these areas.

3.2. Establishing priorities

At this point, it is sensible to evaluate what effect a job change will have on your current lifestyle, financial situation, career path, and relationships. What factors will have the greatest impact on how you choose a new job and protect these interests? Your choices must become even more realistic when you have a wife, children, no second income, student loans to repay, and other such factors.

No working situation is perfect, but you can enhance your chances of being content by identifying the factors that are necessary for you to be an effective employee and to establish a comfort zone in a new position. When evaluating the pros and cons of a job, consider the benefits, location, security, potential, income, and responsibilities.

It has been my experience that these are the factors that most often come to play when a person is considering a new position. Use this list as a guide. Add important factors you find are missing. Then choose the three factors that are most important to you. These will be your top three priorities. Now, whenever possible, do not interview for a position that does not satisfy your top three priorities! Remember, no job is perfect—you are looking for a comfort zone.

4. Conquering the resumé

4.1. *Myths versus truisms: Preparing the resumé*

There are many myths regarding what makes a good resumé:

- Colored paper is better.
- Never fax a resumé, you will look too desperate.
- You need a different resumé for different types of positions.
- The longer the resumé the better.
- Always include a complete list of publications.
- Make it look like you did more than you did. You can learn it later.
- Your experience will look better by presenting class work in a way that makes it look like a job.
- Do not put a job on a resumé if you will get a bad reference.
- Everyone is impressed if you begin by writing an objective.

Colored paper is okay, but some colors do not fax or copy well. Believe it or not, most organizations that are attempting to fill a position will review every resumé submitted. Content will get you a second look, not the color of paper.

In an ideal world, a resumé produced specifically for a particular position would be wonderful! But, do you have this kind of time? Put together a resumé that highlights your most marketable attributes, and make sure you stress accomplishments, not duties. It would be an onerous task for most people to write a different resumé for each job for which they apply, but it might be practical to have one resumé for clinical positions and another for those in academia.

Your resumé should be as concise as possible while still highlighting your professional strengths. Be specific. Listing a series of jobs without dates will telegraph to the interviewer that you lack job stability. Use common acronyms when possible for brevity. For example, rather than "experience with low-dose-rate and high-dose-rate brachytherapy" say "experience with both LDR and HDR brachytherapy." Be specific. If you have observed a procedure as part of a group, say so. If you have hands-on experience with a certain procedure, make that clear. Any experience becomes doubly important when competently performed unsupervised and should be noted on your resumé.

When you consider the effort that goes into preparing a scientific document, it is painful to realize that listing your publications on your resumé might be more harmful than helpful. If your goal is to be a faculty member in a university setting, make sure you include the list of publications and that the list is complete and accurate. However, if your desired position is in a community-based clinical setting, do not list your publications; rather, indicate that a list of publications is available. One of the most common complaints I hear is that PhD medical physicists too often hibernate in their offices staring at a computer screen contemplating research opportunities and that these "computer gazers" lack the communication skills needed to contribute effectively in the clinic setting. So, indicating that you have published large numbers of articles, though admirable, could work to your disadvantage even though you may be completely capable and willing to adapt socially.

Your resumé should describe who you are, not who you want to be. If you try to make undergraduate training appear as postgraduate experience, you will be perceived as dishonest, not experienced. This ruse worked for a few for a while but is now viewed with disdain. You have a responsibility as a professional caregiver to be honest about your background. A discussion of references follows in Section 5, "References."

A written objective at the beginning of a resumé helps only if your objective exactly fits the job for which you are applying. If your stated goal is different, a well-meaning human resources representative may place your resumé in the stack of unsuitables. Perhaps this is one section of the resumé were customization might be feasible; otherwise, I believe that an objective is best omitted.

There are a great number of books in the library on resumé formats. Make sure that you choose one that deals with resumés aimed at technical positions. Keep your resumé simple and to the point, and remember to stress accomplishments rather than duties. It is okay to eliminate some information because of federal statutes. Guidelines set by the Equal Employment Opportunity Commission and numerous other federal agencies say that you do not need to indicate your age, marital status, or whether you are challenged by a physical disability when writing a resumé. Although it is not mandatory, I suggest that you indicate your citizenship or immigration status if there is going to be any doubt. It is federally regulated that employers verify your legal status regarding employment before they hire you. Advising potential employers of your immigration status in the resumé might prevent a lost interviewing opportunity.

4.2. Distributing your resumé

Now that you have this powerful resumé, whom do you give it to? The answer will depend on the stage of your career. New graduates will want to start with any professional contacts they have made. An experienced applicant should forward a resumé to the potential employer, if his or her background meets the qualifications of a particular job listing. The most frequent complaint from organizations about responses to the American Association of Physicists in Medicine job listings is that a tremendous number of respondents are not qualified for a position but respond anyway. Read job listings carefully, and make sure you qualify before responding.

Professional recruiters are an excellent resource for the job hunter with experience. See Section 7, "Working with a "headhunter," for details about this approach.

5. References

Collect as many reference contacts as you can, but use them judiciously, and always obtain permission! As a new graduate, your reference contacts will be your instructors and anyone you might have worked with or for. Later, your reference contacts will be someone who has actual knowledge of your work performance, character, and interpersonal skills. Beware of two pitfalls. First, do not abuse the goodwill of a reference contact, especially one that you value highly. Are you really interested in this position or is it just 1 of 15 you have applied for? Is the job really worth the telephone call that might be made to your reference contact? Second, make sure the person you indicate as a reference contact will speak favorably of you; otherwise, you will have created a problem for yourself. The responses I regret most when I call a reference contact are "Is this confidential?" or "Will you tell (the applicant) what I say?" According to the Fair Credit Reporting Act of 1970, the applicant has a legal right to the contents of the conversation between a hiring authority or interviewer and the specified reference contact. To obtain a copy of the content of the reference, the applicant would need only to write a letter to the hiring authority or interviewer who obtained the reference and ask for a copy. If the reference contact asks, he or she must be informed of the applicant's right, and the applicant must be given a copy of the reference if it is requested.

A good rule to follow is three great references are better than seven mediocre ones. Conversely, you do need to provide an adequate choice of reference contacts. However, do not send a list of reference contacts with a resumé when responding to an advertisement. Reserve you best ammunition until you are sure the organization has an interest in you and vice versa.

Your resumé should indicate that references are available upon request. When possible, reserve letters of reference for presentation at a follow-up to the initial interview. If sent to the most influential person, your name and background will remain on their minds for a long period of time, which will enhance your chances of being considered

6. Networking

Pardon me if this particular line of rhetoric has become tiresome, but never underestimate the power of your network. If three people each tell three other people about you and these three people each tell three other people…well, you see the point. Always use your personal network to help find a good job. It is a truism that many times it is not what you know but who you know. Let's assume that you have just graduated. You have impressed your advisors and instructors. They are impressed or you would not have been successful in graduate school, especially at your institution, right? Ask for help!

One Saturday I was caught in traffic at an intersection where a group of youngsters were raising money by washing cars. I had had my automobile washed earlier in the day, and it was obvious that it did not need cleaning. One child motioned persistently for me to roll down my window. When I finally obliged, the young man maybe 9 or 10 years old, poked his head in the window and said, "Lady, we take donations!" Laughing, I gave him some dollar bills while wishing I had more. What a salesperson or politician he will make! That child had learned, at a tender age, a lesson that many of us never learn. You have to ask for what you want. This example illustrates that you may accomplish a great deal through your particular network, but you will need to make the first step: asking for assistance. "I need a job. Who do you know who might need a person of my background?"

7. Working with a "headhunter"

The professional "headhunter" (or recruiter) will be able to help you assess your value, critique your resumé, prepare for an interview, and negotiate for salary and benefits. The most valuable assets of a full-time recruiter are: 1) their knowledge of your area of expertise and the organizations that hire people like you and 2) their time. Sending a resumé to the wrong "headhunter" could be the worst thing possible. There are several potentially harmful behaviors perpetrated by unethical recruiters that you should know about. Recruiters are ethically restricted from sending resumés to an organization with whom they do not have a contract. Nonetheless, a dishonest recruiter who happens upon the resumé of a highly qualified candidate may forward an unsolicited resumé to an organization needing a medical physicist anyway. This puts the applicant at a disadvantage, because the organization may not accept the resumé from the recruiter and may not accept a resumé later sent directly by the applicant. Find out what organizations a particular recruiter has contracts with. Another unethical recruiting practice is that some recruiters will "shotgun" resumés to a long list of companies hoping that one will fall into the hands of a human resources representative responsible for filling a medical physics position. Sadly, this approach has resulted in a person's resumé being sent to their current employer!

Some recruiters will misrepresent a job even when they know that problems exist. An ethical recruiter will tell the applicant about the problems associated with a given position as well as the perks, even if the candidate insists on pursuing the job.

There was a position at an organization on the East Coast that involved so many problems that a group of the medical physicists who had worked there formed a club and met once a month to compare notes on the latest alarming story about the job. Some of these medical physicists had been placed at the organization by recruiters who neglected to tell them that the physician they did not meet during the interview was loud, verbally abusive, and unreasonable. I know the two medical physicists who hold the record for the shortest and longest times spent in this position. One board-certified medical physicist lasted 2 weeks in the position before he quit in disgust. Another, a very forgiving individual, held the position for 3 years. He was rewarded for his service by being fired without cause or notice. I am aware of at least five others who have worked in the position in the last 6 years, including the one who worked there for 3 whole years. Would I ever send someone to interview there? Only if the abusive physician left. Will some recruiters send people there to interview before the physician leaves even though they are aware of the problems? Yes.

An ethical recruiter will tell you the truth. A truly good recruiter will find out what problems exist in a job and tell you about them. An exceptional recruiter will try to educate the people responsible for hiring about potential problems at their organization before a search begins. Once in a while, problems are solved before the interviews begin.

Ultimately, employing the talents of a recruiter is a real-life game of "Whom do I trust?" Here is an area where networking can be of great value. Ask friends, business associates, or professors for a recommendation for a recruiter. It is important that you identify a headhunter with whom you can communicate and whose judgment you trust.

In this commentary, I have constantly urged you to network. A survey conducted by Drake Beam Morin, Inc., and reported in *What Color is Your Parachute* by Richard Bolles (1970) reported a 15% success rate among applicants who use search firms. Of those surveyed:

* 68% found employment through personal contacts
* 15% found employment through a search firm's activities
* 9% found employment by responding to help wanted ads
* 8% found employment by mass mailing their resumé, an employment letter, or both

Once you find a recruiter you can trust, be honest with him or her about your background, experience, and goals. Recruiters are hired to find individuals with a specific skill set—not trainees. A recruiter can help you only if your skill set is in demand and he or she knows what you do, how to evaluate your skills, and where the good positions are. The recruiter's client is the organization—not the applicant. The organization pays the recruiter to find a qualified person for a specific job. The recruiter knows, however, that an unhappy employee probably will not do a very good job and that it is in everyone's best interest that the applicant also be happy. Be aware of the lines of responsibility and loyalty when working with a recruiter.

8. The interview

You must prepare for an interview much like you would a final exam. Preparation for a final exam begins at the start of the semester. Preparation for an interview should begin with a realistic analysis of who you are and the recognition of those intrinsic qualities that will allow you to succeed.

8.1. Dress to impress

The first lesson is dress the part. Everyone else might be in blue jeans and lab coats, but the interviewee must be dressed to impress. As described in Section 2.3, "Personal presentation," your goal should be to project a clean, tidy, conservative look; nothing flashy, revealing, or suggestive; nothing that would leave a lasting, negative image. Whatever you choose to wear, make sure that you feel good about how you look. If you are satisfied with your appearance, you will exude an air of confidence that will positively impact the interview.

8.2. Be your most pleasant self

There is no substitute for enthusiasm and interest. Both are flattering to the interviewer. If you also happen to be talented, you gain additional approval points. An aloof, superior attitude is unacceptable interview behavior. You have not done the organization a favor by being there, but they might have a tremendous impact on your future. You need to let them know that what they have to offer is important to you!

Everyone you meet during an on-site visit is important. The secretary you were rude to before just might have input in the hiring decision. The new therapist might say something agreeable about you, if you were cordial to him. If you are the quiet type, be quiet. If you are outgoing, be outgoing. Be yourself, but be your nicest most positive self.

8.3. Bring along pertinent data, just in case

You may or may not be asked to fill out an application during the visit, but count on having to do that at some point in the interviewing process. Be prepared. Make sure you have the appropriate information with you: full and correct names, telephone numbers, and addresses of former employees, supervisors, references, etc. This is not a situation where you should borrow a directory. You must fill out the application completely. Writing "see resume" on any portion of an application is unacceptable. Filling out the paperwork may be tiresome but filling it out completely is mandatory. The people at that hiring institution know how the application is designed, and they can find information about you in a hurry when they need it. Make it easy for them. You may also want to take along a couple of extra copies of your resume. Do not hand them out willy-nilly, but have them on hand just in case. If you are fresh out of a residency program, consider taking along some copies of your work, for example, samples of machine calibrations or dosimetry plans. When using dosimetry plans, make sure that the patient's name is obliterated. Even if you are newly graduated, there will be someone at the organization who will appreciate your work; if not, you probably should not be interviewing there in the first place, right?

8.4. *Your body language speaks volumes*

Your handshake should be a firm greeting, not a wrestling feat. Look people in the eyes when you speak to them. Looking away in the middle of an answer implies that you could be unsure or lying. It is fine to look down, up, or to the side when contemplating an answer but not in the middle of responding. You do not need to sit or stand at attention during the interview, but do not get too relaxed either. Be alert, look and act interested, and listen closely.

8.5. *You think you heard what you thought I said…*

Listening can be a difficult and exhausting task, but it is never more essential than during an interview. It is crucial for you to understand a question before you supply an answer. If the question is vague, ask a clarifying question. One of my least favorite non-questions is "Tell me about yourself." What an opportunity to say something absolutely wrong. Your great Aunt Edith may have been the single most important influence in your life, but the interviewer probably does not really care about dear Aunt Edith. So, amplify the question! To the non-question "Tell me about yourself" say "Sure, what would you like to know?" In response to "Tell me about M. D. Anderson" reply "Certainly, from what point of view?" Make sure that you tell them what they really want to know by answering the correct question.

8.6. *Be prepared for the hot-seat questions*

The most commonly asked interview questions are "What are your strengths?" and "What are you weaknesses?" During your first few contacts with the hospital or clinic, find out why the position you are applying for is open and the nature of the organization's biggest problem. Once you know these things and if you have already prepared a feature/benefit presentation, you can tailor your response to the first question (about strengths) so that you appear well-informed and confident. When you are fully cognizant of your benefit to the workforce at large, you can easily point out how your strengths will be of value to that particular organization. Present yourself as a solution to their problems whenever possible.

Figure out what your greatest weakness is and how you would improve that aspect of your personality. Tell a future employer about your greatest weakness only if you are pretty sure it will show up on a reference from a previous employer. Be truthful when answering this question, but you do not need to tell them everything your mother or closest friend knows. Whenever possible, claim as a weakness a trait the employer will actually find admirable. For example, saying "I am a workaholic" would not exactly displease a potential employer. Are you too picky where your calibrations are concerned? Please ask one of your reference contacts to state that as one of your weaknesses! Where flaws are concerned, be honest, but only mention one or two and choose these carefully.

Some other standard interview questions you might expect are:

- What do you know about our organization?
- Why did you become a medical physicist?
- Career-wise, where do you want to be in 5 years?
- What kind of a boss are you looking for?
- Describe your least favorite place to work?
- Why did you leave your previous job?
- What kind of relationship do you expect to have with a dosimetrist? an administrator? a radiation oncologist?
- What is the most difficult thing you have ever had to do?
- Do you think you can do this job? Why?

Once again, prepare for an interview as you would for a final exam. I urge you to actually write down answers to some of these questions and become comfortable reciting the answers out loud. The more you prepare the better you will do. Scrutinize the interviewing organization as best you can. One advantage to working with a good recruiter is his or her knowledge of the industry. Your recruiter should be able to give you background information about the organization you are interviewing with. You should also network on your own. Ask people you know about the organization. Someone will know someone who will know someone else who works there or did work there.

8.7. Your turn to ask the questions

There are some areas that should never be explored during an interview. For example, never ask a question that in any way implies "What is this organization going to do for me?" Rather, ask about the position you are applying for, the structure of the organization, why the job is available, what the organization wants to accomplished in the next 6 months, what their biggest challenge has been, etc. You might even ask the interviewer what he or she likes about working for the organization themselves. Again, be interested, enthusiastic, and eager. Avoid questions about benefits, salary, vacation, meeting expenses, raises, and adding additional staff. However, once you are offered a position and before you accept it, ask about each and every one of these things.

A word of caution: Never, ever say anything negative about your most recent employer. It is a weird mental twist, but if you speak poorly of a previous employer, the interviewer will turn that around in his mind and remember the negatives you say as if you said them about him.

One last but important suggestion about the interview: If you want the job, ask for it! As I keep saying, there is no substitute for interest and enthusiasm. If you experience a successful interview, you will increase your chances of receiving an offer by 60% if you ask for the job. Be careful, though. Know exactly what you are going to say. Practice asking for the job aloud. Formulate the words before you walk into the interview. You might say "Mr. Employer, I am exceptionally impressed with your clinic and the staff. I feel I could offer a great deal to this organization and I hope to receive an offer." Or say "Mr. Jones, I would really like to work here. When will you decide whom to hire?" Pushy? Probably. Necessary? Absolutely!

8.8. Negotiating salary and benefits in the interview

If you are asked about your salary requirements during the interview, be straight-forward and honest, but avoid saying anything that would be binding. For example, say "Mr. Interviewer, I hesitate to give you a dollar figure. Like most people, I want the most money possible, but I want this job! Any dollar figure I say could either be too high or too low. Because of that, I would really appreciate knowing what you have in mind for me." Or "I would really appreciate the opportunity to consider your best offer." Or "Great! I would love to work here! What dollar figure did you have in mind!" You can always refuse an offer but you cannot say "Only kidding" after you determine that the dollar amount you spontaneously came up with is $8,000 more than their maximum or $5,000 less than their minimum.

In some cases, there is a comfortable trade-off between salary and benefits. In other cases, the benefits are not very good. Once again, decide before the interview what you must have and what is a "throw away." A knowledgeable recruiter will be of great assistance during these times. He or she can ask questions that might be awkward for you without jeopardizing your offer.

If you are not offered the position at the conclusion of the interview, ask the interviewer when they plan to make a decision. If a decision date has not been chosen or they seem unwilling to give a definite date, ask when it would be appropriate for you to call them back. That way, you have a semi-appointment to call back, and you can feel comfortable doing so.

9. You want how much money?

At some point in your career, you may be successful enough and lucky enough to dictate your salary. Until then, however, you might want to consider some basic economic factors. Review your priorities. What is the most important consideration at this point in your career? When I ask people why they want to change jobs, money is rarely the answer, although money is certainly important when a job change is made. In most instances, the impetus to look is supplied by something else.

When assessing your salary requirements, use the 20th, 50th, and 80th percentiles at the appropriate years of experience from the American Association of Physicists in

Medicine salary survey. The mean salary overly weights very high salaries of a few and is not particularly useful. In any event, you can usually count on inadequate wages for your first position. Depending on opportunities in the area of the country where you prefer to live, this low-paid status could continue from 2 to 5 years or until you become board certified. It is a universal truth that professionals developing a career path usually change jobs in the early years as a means to advance their way up the salary ladder.

Many variables contribute to the actual benefit you will receive from a given dollar figure. You need to be particularly aware of the cost of living for any location. For instance, Texas is one of eight states that does not have a state income tax. But when you compare Texas' property taxes with those of other states, the advantage of no state income tax dims. Living in paradise likewise has its price. When a particular locale is in demand, salaries go down. In 1997, the state of Colorado was one of the most notable examples of this dilemma. North Carolina followed at a close second. When comparing the value of a dollar with the allure of a popular location, realize that the smaller, more out of the way the town is, the greater the potential to earn a higher salary because there will be fewer physicists to compete with.

Decide what will make you happiest. What type of weather can you and your family least tolerate—the heat, the cold, or humidity? Do you prefer flatlands or mountains, big cities or suburban settings? Realistically distinguish your "wants" from your actual "needs" and "desires." Do not make a decision about a job or a salary offer based on a wish list; instead, base your decision on a thoughtful assessment of yourself and your situation. Remain aware of motivational factors, but remember to keep your choices in perspective. Follow patterns that will allow you to be content until the situation becomes more favorable. You may have to drown in humidity in a rural community and accept a lower salary until you gain enough experience to assume a role of greater responsibility in an exciting urban area earning top-notch pay. In the meantime, be as flexible as possible, and remember that what your former college roommate "says" he or she is making is just that—what they "say".

10. Conclusion

Be assured that at some point in your future, all of the preparation and analysis suggested here will help in the development of a career that is challenging but carries great satisfaction. The keys to a successful job search/personal marketing plan are to be prepared; project a confident, enthusiastic attitude; know what you have to offer (features) and how you can help the organization achieve its goals (benefits); and make good use of your most important resource, your personal contacts.

References

Bollos RN (1970) What color is your parachute? Berkley, CA:Ten Speed Press

Barbara Walters, BSc

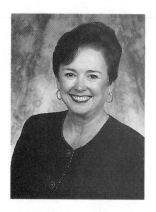

Barbara Walters graduated with bachelor degrees in sociology and social work from the University of Oklahoma in 1968. Ms. Walters has been a recruiter since 1976, having worked for Management Recruiters of Oklahoma City since 1986. Her recruiting specialties are radiation and medical oncology, and she recruits personnel at all levels within a cancer center, from radiotherapy technologists to center administrators. In 1990, Ms. Walters received her accreditation as a Certified Senior Account Manager, and in 1996, she was named one of Management Recruiters Top Ten Account Executives in the Southwest Region of the United States. Ms. Walters is an associate member of the AAPM, and since 1996 has served on an AAPM task group to explore writing a job description for medical physicists.

Professional Job Skills

Your First Job as a Clinical Medical Physicist

Ronald W. Cowart, MS

Memorial Health System of East Texas, Lufkin, TX

Abstract. Your first job as a medical physicist and how to use it to advance your career goals is one of the most significant decisions you will ever make. In targeting your first job, you must assess your skills and define your short-term goals. You must also understand the pros and cons of different opportunities in the medical physics marketplace. Short-term priorities should emphasize gaining experience, not salary. Also, there are several methods key to getting the most out of your first job. Lastly, special skills, continuing education, and networking are essential in advancing one's career. Guidelines for each of these topics are presented here based on my experiences.

1. Introduction

Your first job can be a very satisfying experience. This chapter provides you with a step-by-step guide for making that experience happen. Topics discussed here include assessing your skills, defining and meeting your short-term goals, accepting the right job offer, transitioning from graduate student to employee, meeting the demands of the job, and setting long-term goals for achieving a successful career. Although these topics are illustrated for the therapeutic radiological physicist, the area in which I am board certified, they can be equally applied to all disciplines of medical physics.

2. Taking stock of your skills

An honest assessment of the skills you have developed in medical physics is your first order of business in charting the course you will follow from here. You are undoubtedly strong in some areas and weak in others. Examine what you do best, what you enjoy doing, and what you are willing to do. Consider your capabilities outside the arena of physics. Organizational, leadership, and business skills should be included in your evaluation. This assessment will help you set short-term goals and determine the direction to take in pursuing your career in medical physics.

3. Defining your short-term goals

Long before the interviews begin and before job offers start rolling in, you must devote some time to setting some short-term goals. With these goals in place, the path to a satisfying and productive career is much easier and clearer. The short-term goals that follow are examples that are meant to stimulate you as you set your own personal goals.

3.1. Clinical experience

You need practical clinical experience to complement your graduate-level education. Mastery in the areas of machine commissioning, treatment planning, quality-assurance, and physician/patient consultation are prerequisites to a successful career whether or not you decide to stay in the clinic as part of a long-term goal. There is no substitute for work experience in the clinical environment. Physicians, therapists, technologists, and dosimetrists all look to the physicist for answers to difficult problems in and out of the clinic.

3.2. Board certification

An important short-term goal in your budding career is to become board certified. Our field has rapidly become one in which board certification is required for employment. A workplace in which you perform under the supervision of a broad-certified medical physicist is a prerequisite to certification; so, your job search should include a search for a good mentor. A mentor can help you assemble the skills needed to pass the certification examination as quickly as possible. The mentor should be able to put you on the fast track to the certification process. There are many more opportunities and higher compensation available for a board-certified medical physicist. I strongly encourage you to make certification one of the highest priorities among your short-term goals.

3.3. Strong work ethic

Strive to develop a reputation for honesty, integrity, and hard work. Such a reputation is fashioned over time; it cannot be purchased, it must be earned. Integrity means doing the right thing, even if it is unpopular, unfashionable, and unprofitable. Draw a solid ethical line and never cross it. Do not cut corners in the workplace, and be prepared to stay until your work is complete. Make good on your promises; if you are not sure you can deliver, do not make the promise in the first place. If you find yourself in a situation where you are unsure, listen to your conscience. Do not perform work you are not qualified nor competent to perform unsupervised. Lastly, always seek the good in others, and they will more likely find good in you.

3.4. Interpersonal skills

Interpersonal skills go a long way toward determining how easily your career track unfolds. These skills are very important yet often overlooked in our profession. Set a goal to become accomplished in interpersonal interactions by considering the following:

- Practice being a good listener. Talk 20% of the time, and listen 80%. When someone is relating a story, do not interrupt with a story of your own.

- Take every opportunity to praise others for their successes, both business and personal. Take the time to compliment someone when they deserve it. Be the person in your office who makes everyone smile. Everyone loves a cheerful person and looks forward to seeing them.

- Do not be confrontational. If someone is confrontational with you, avoid a response. The next day is always a better time to deal with a confrontational individual. Most will regret their actions given time to reflect. People who can hold their tongue rarely have any trouble holding their friends.

- Do not be a complainer. Every department has one, do not let it be you. When others begin to criticize, fight the urge to join the slaughter. Look for solutions, not problems. Anyone can identify problems.

- Be a team player. Reject attempts to put fellow employees in a pecking order. Treat all employees with respect and dignity. Their jobs are as important to them as yours is to you.

4. Reviewing the different opportunities in the job market

The workplace environment in which you may find yourself will vary from a one-stop, one-person physics show at a small hospital to a 50-person physics staff at a large academic institution. Each type of workplace has advantages and disadvantages as a first job site.

4.1. One-person department

This workplace environment is an excellent place to quickly hone your clinical skills. After all, the physicist usually performs all functions required of a physics staff, including dosimetry, quality assurance, and radiation safety. It is easy to get an overall perspective of how the clinic works because this medical physicist is usually very busy doing it all, and thus, is looking for an assistant. This is probably your quickest route to gaining the experience you require.

However, there are some potential disadvantages to working in this environment. First, this physicist will be your only contact. If your personalities conflict or if he or she is not keen on helping you gain experience, then you will be thwarted in your efforts to advance. Second, a small hospital does not purchase new equipment very often. It may be 10 years between major purchases of linacs, simulators, and treatment-planning computers. This means you may never experience machine commissioning or treatment-planning computer commissioning, both of which provide you with extremely valuable experience. Finally, a small hospital is not likely to provide manpower-intensive services such as stereotactic irradiation, total-skin irradiation, and three-dimensional treatment planning; instead, they will refer those cases to larger hospitals that can achieve economies of scale for these types of treatments.

Notwithstanding the above points, a good mentor at a small hospital provides you with a learning experience that is hard to beat.

4.2. Larger university hospital

This workplace environment will likely have many accelerators, simulators, and treatment-planning computers as well as an active program of research. You will be exposed to a variety of equipment here, a definite plus. Also, your department is very likely to commission equipment while you are employed there, another great opportunity for you. Additionally, there will likely be a full complement of services offered, including stereotactic, total-skin, and three-dimensional treatment planning. You will likely find other personnel near your level of experience with whom you can network.

The opportunities at an institution of this size are boundless, but there also are numerous pitfalls that can snare you on your path to gaining experience here. Large university hospitals tend to be very compartmentalized and specialized. There will most likely be separate sections in the department for dosimetry, quality assurance, machine commissioning, new technology, research, and other areas. You are much more likely to be pigeonholed in a very specific job under these conditions. Your exposure to the overall functions of the clinic will be limited. It takes much more individual effort on your part to get the overall experience you need here. You will have to voluntarily interact with multiple personnel to get the experience and knowledge you require. Your acquisition of experience will typically be slower here than in a smaller workplace, but broader in scope.

4.3. Medical physics group

These groups offer service to multiple radiotherapy clinics. The service provided by this group can range from a 1-day a week visit to full-time staffing by one or several medical physicists. In this environment, the group is most often looking for a medical physicist who can function independently at one or several clinics. You will not yet be qualified to assume this type of position. Occasionally, however, a service group may require a medical physicist to work in a setting with other medical physicists full time. This is the type of situation in which you may be interested, because it offers a similar environment to that of the one-man department but provides a better opportunity to interact with multiple medical physicists and use different types of equipment. Service groups accepting you for your first job are often motivated to train you rapidly as it translates directly to their bottom line. This can make for a rewarding and exciting first job.

4.4. Radiological Physics Center

A unique opportunity exists for the first-time job applicant who can secure a position with the Radiological Physics Center (RPC) located at The University of Texas M. D.

97

Anderson Cancer Center in Houston, TX. This group, under the guidance of the Radiation Therapy Committee of the American Association of Physicists in Medicine, is charged with assessing the accuracy of radiation dose delivered to patients at radiotherapy facilities participating in National Cancer Institute clinical trails. To accomplish this goal, the RPC must send a medical physicist to each participating center periodically. The RPC physicist does a mini-commissioning of each machine in the center. Additionally, the RPC physicist must review the dosimetry calculation system in place at the center to understand how it is applied. Charts of patients at the center who complete their protocol treatment are sent to the RPC for review. There, the charts are checked for accuracy of final tumor dose. The data and information the RPC medical physicist gathered during the visit to that center are used to make this assessment. This job exposes you to a variety of equipment, methods, and personnel. You benefit from seeing how radiotherapy is practiced at multiple centers, and you meet a variety of medical physicists. This experience is invaluable as you set long-term goals and are able to select which of these workplaces has the conditions you most enjoy. The downside to working for the RPC is the relatively little treatment-planning experience you acquire and the nonexistent patient contact and clinic experience. This experience must be garnered elsewhere.

5. Getting the job you want

The resumé writing, interviewing, and negotiating process is discussed in more detail in the chapter entitled, "The Job Search and Marketing Yourself," by Barbara Walters. However, keep a few points in mind as you acquire that first position. Focus on the potential jobs that best satisfy your short-term goals. Remember that meeting the short-term goals is far more important than commanding a premium salary. You will have plenty of opportunity to achieve the salary level you desire once you have met your short-term goals. Definitely negotiate for salary, but do not make it a primary focus. It is much more important at this stage of your career to negotiate for experience! It is hard to resist the temptation to go for the highest paying position, particularly when it is your first real job. Be patient and explore all the nuances of any job offered, and you will be better off. In a tight job market, it is better to accept peanuts for wages and gain much-needed experience than to hold out a year or more for higher wages.

6. From the university to your first job

6.1. The first 2 weeks and orientation

When starting a new job, particularly a first job, you will be filled with anxiety and doubt. Take it a step at a time, and the road will be smooth. Begin by allowing yourself some time and space to ease into your first job. You are not expected to know it all on your first day. Plan on devoting the first week to a structured orientation process. Whether or not your organization provides a formal orientation, make time to orient yourself to the administration of your organization. Find out who to ask for help and who the key people in your organization are. If you are not introduced to these people, introduce yourself. Familiarize yourself with the policy and procedure manuals for your organization and your department. Take the time now to clarify your role and duties and your supervisor's expectations. Find out who will supervise your efforts and how closely your work will be reviewed. You need to feel comfortable with the amount of responsibility you are given. It is important at this stage of your career to have close supervision and feedback while performing in the clinic. Ask lots of questions and observe how things are done. Now is not the time to be shy.

6.2. Performing your duties

Working in a new clinical position always has a steep learning curve. The pace for the first few weeks of employment is quite hectic. The transition is made more difficult because things are usually done quite differently in your workplace than in the radiation therapy department in which you trained. There is equipment that will be new to you. Personnel are likely to have different responsibilities than you expect. Calculation methods and recordkeeping will almost certainly be different. Remember: the way you learned to practice clinical physics is not the only way. Be flexible, inquisitive, and attentive. You gain a great deal of experience by just understanding how different clinics do their business. There are multiple methods of arriving at the end point of delivering radiation accurately to the patient.

After a few weeks on your new job, the hectic pace of accumulating information, fitting in, and learning new ways will slow down. After getting the feel of your new job, doubts and anxieties begin to subside as you move from an orientation process to accomplishing your job responsibilities. You now have a clear picture of what you are expected to do. You can focus on performing your assigned duties in a timely, efficient, and consistent manner. Strive to be the first to arrive at work or the last to leave. Develop a reputation for performing an honest day's work. Start to focus on a timeline to meet your short-term goals in your new position. Keep an open line of communication with your medical physicist supervisor who will serve as an immensely valuable asset to you. Ask your supervisor if it would be possible to have weekly meetings for your first several months of employment to make sure you are on the right track with your job and your short-term goals. Explain to the supervisor that you want to maximize your strengths and minimize any weaknesses related to your experience by turning them into strengths. Add that you are prepared to do whatever it takes to accomplish your goal of becoming a productive team player. Follow-up on any suggestions and advice the supervisor may give you and relate these facts back to him or her. Be sure to thank the supervisor for assisting you.

6.3. Two months down the road

After your first several months of meetings have ended, thank your supervisor for helping you succeed in you new job. Volunteer for every project that the two of you agree will be a career-broadening experience or would aid you in getting board certified. Tell your supervisor that you are so appreciative of the help you have received so far that you would like to continue the process by sitting down once a month and reviewing your progress and plans and getting feedback on your performance. Several interesting things will happen when you take this approach. You will be the beneficiary of a great deal of one-on-one attention and positive feedback, not to mention the possibility of exposure to important information that might not otherwise come your way. A supervisor approached in this way will more times than not befriend you and readily help such an eager learner achieve goals. An additional benefit will be realized at performance review time. Once a year, prior to any salary increase, you will be given an annual performance review in a meeting with your supervisor who often knows little or nothing about the actual quality of your work. The strategy outlined here will give you the added benefit of meeting with the supervisor one-on-one at least 12 times more frequently than any other employee. I guarantee this person will be one of your lifelong supporters and a great reference if you will follow this advice. The importance of networking skills such as these in the small community of medical physics cannot be stressed enough. The good jobs in this field rarely make it to the monthly placement bulletin published by the American Association of Physicists in Medicine. Instead, they are filled through networking with other medical physicists.

7. Job security

You will hear the term "job security" bantered about often in the workplace. In point of fact, the only job security you will ever have sits between your ears. You cannot be assured, whatever is promised, that you will always maintain the position you now occupy. In a time of rapid technological and economic change in the medical field, your security with any one particular employer cannot be guaranteed. Your job security will come from the development of skills in a broad variety of areas intended to complement your medical physics skills.

8. Achieving success

8.1. Broaden your skills

Computer skills are indispensable in our profession. Whether performing clinical or administrative duties, you must be computer literate. Goals here should include proficiency in at least one programming language, such as FORTRAN, Pascal, Basic, or C++. The newer PC-based visual languages are also excellent tools. Visual Basic, Visual C++, and Delphi are extremely good tools for producing quick solutions to everyday problems. An absolute requirement here is to learn a spreadsheet language inside and out. Excel and Lotus 123 are good examples. You should be able to program fluently in their macro languages. Spreadsheet programs have become amazingly productive tools for accomplished users. Examples of spreadsheet applications in medical physics include speedy data charting and graphing with minimal effort, completely automated data acquisition systems, brilliant quality assurance tools, and monitor-unit calculation programs. Knowledge of networks also is a worthwhile asset. Pick up a few books on networks and begin reading. A good grounding in computer skills will quickly become one of your most valuable skills. These skills are in constant demand in all work environments.

Become an expert in the billing aspects of your profession. Become familiar with the charge-capture process at your workplace. Educate yourself about Current Procedural Terminology (CPT) codes and how you should bill those codes in your workplace. Know what the radiation oncologists should bill and how they bill. The radiation oncology billing process is complicated, and it is often misinterpreted. It takes a substantial amount of effort to fully understand and apply billing for maximum reimbursement by Medicare, private insurance companies, and managed-care companies. An amazing number of workplaces do not bill all the procedures possible nor do they bill correctly. You will get high marks from your administration for staying on top of the ever-changing billing process. Such knowledge also will contribute to your bottom line. Give it some attention.

8.2. Continue your education

Make learning a lifelong vocation. What you learn will affect what you earn. Stay on top of developments in medical physics. Do not retreat from education because you feel secure and comfortable. Technology and change are inevitable. Stay on the cutting edge in all your fields of expertise. Challenge yourself so as not to become complacent. Remember that your job security ultimately depends on your expertise.

8.3. Maintain a network

The importance of maintaining a network of contacts and friendships in your profession has already been alluded to in this article. Again, the importance of such a network cannot be emphasized enough. As you progress through your career, you will notice a common thread in all top-notch people. They seem to know all the other really top-notch people in their field or can reach them with several phone calls. The top people in every field have made a long-term, concerted effort to communicate with and learn from their peers. You will almost certainly meet these people through affiliation with the American Association of Physicists in Medicine, the American College of Medical Physics, the American College of Radiology, and other professional societies. Maintain your professional memberships; they are important vehicles in your networking efforts.

Networking within your hospital and community is just as important. Medical physics is not a well-understood profession. It will be up to you to educate your administration and community regarding your skills. Volunteer to assist your administration with radiation safety issues and any technology-related problems they face. A well-rounded physicist often brings more to the table than any other hospital staff member with respect to technological problems. Join your local Rotary or Lions

Club. This is a particularly valuable network in a smaller community. Do not let the lawyers, doctors, and other businessmen dictate the professional environment of your community. Extend the visibility of your profession by offering your comments to newspaper and TV reporters in your hometown or suburban community when sensational headlines occur. You can often give them a clear and concise picture of the truth and fiction in one of those reports about radon, nuclear meltdown, cellular phones causing brain cancer, or electrical highlines causing leukemia.

Network, network, network! You cannot have too many friends.

References

American Medical Association (1997) Current Procedural Terminology. Chicago, IL: AMA

Ronald W. Cowart, MS

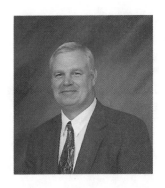

Ronald Cowart received his master's of science degree in Biomedical Science (Medical Physics) from The University of Texas Graduate School of Biomedical Sciences in Houston, TX in 1976. From 1976 to1981, he worked in the Section of Diagnostic Radiology Physics in the Department of Physics at The University of Texas M. D. Anderson Cancer Center, Houston, TX. He then joined the Radiological Physics Center, where he worked from 1981 to 1982. In 1983, he worked as a medical physicist at The University of Texas Medical Branch in Galveston, TX. In late 1983, Mr. Cowart returned to M. D. Anderson Cancer Center to work on reengineering of the cyclotron. In 1987, he became Director of Radiation Physics Engineering Services, supervising cyclotron and accelerator maintenance, shop services, and engineering services in the Department of Radiation Physics. In 1989, Mr. Cowart became a consulting medical physicist at Arthur Temple Cancer Center in Lufkin, TX, where he became Cancer Center Director in 1997. In 1998, Mr. Cowart became a Vice President and Chief Information Officer of the Memorial Health System of East Texas, a network of five hospitals in the East Texas region. He is responsible for strategic planning for technology development in his role as Chief Information Officer. He retains responsibility as a consulting medical physicist to the cancer center there. Mr. Cowart has had the unique experience of having worked as a medical physicist in small, medium, and large radiation oncology clinics. His job responsibilities have ranged from very specific duties in quality assurance and engineering support to the very broad responsibility of being the single medical physicist. His unique experiences make him very aware of the wide range of expectations of the clinical medical physicist.

Interacting with Administrators

Michael D. Mills, PhD

Radiation Oncology Department, University of Louisville, Brown Cancer Center, Louisville, KY

Abstract. The prospect of negotiating with an administrator requires the medical physicist to think carefully about a number of issues and then to document these thoughts. Whose interests do I serve? To whom do I properly report with respect to the various facets of my employment? What rules exist and what sanctions are in place if I break the rules? What do I ultimately intend to accomplish? The medical physicist should also consider how the administrator would answer these questions. The negotiation process is simplified if the medical physicist and administrator agree on the professional framework and role of the medical physicist on the health care team. The medical physicist must identify his or her essential interests and determine in advance a plan to meet not only these interests but also those of the administrator. The goal is to reach an agreement that will preserve the interests of both parties and maintain the relationship. As employment satisfaction depends largely on the outcome of such a negotiation, it is essential for the medical physicist to spend some time mastering the skill of negotiation. Peace of mind results from the assurance that "I have done my very best for myself and my family."

1. Introduction

The changes brought about by managed care have caused great uncertainty for upper-level health care managers. The costs are high for acquisition and operation of emerging technologies such as picture archiving and communications systems, digital radiology, magnetic resonance imaging, three-dimensional (3-D) conformal radiotherapy, intensity-modulated radiotherapy (IMRT), and many others. Questions that managers must address include: Does this technology benefit the patient? Does the benefit justify the cost? Who will utilize these services, and how will they be used? What will happen if the acquisition is deferred? Is acquisition of this technology necessary to compete for managed-care contracts? What personnel resources at what expense must be devoted to this new service? Radiation oncology physics services account for 30% or more of the cost of radiation oncology. In many cases, the manager struggles to understand the technology well enough to direct those who actually perform the work. Here, accurate and verifiable information is key. When a manager is faced with a new situation, the first response is predictable: A telephone call is placed to a colleague who may have faced the situation already. However, the quality and value of information acquired in this manner is subject to question. Are the situations truly comparable? Is the technology truly the same between various vendors? Are the personnel resources truly comparable? What level of control does the manager have over the situation? What level of control does he need?

In many cases, the manager is responsible for bringing new services to the community but has only limited authority. So, the manager learns to manage in situations that do not command authority, and is neither controlled nor controlling. Although management textbooks still talk mainly about managing subordinates, health professionals are no longer evaluated in terms of how many people they supervise. That standard does not mean as much as the complexity of the job, the information used and generated, and the different kinds of relationships needed to do the work.

This observation cuts two ways for medical physicists. First, the medical physicist is often asked to manage technologists, therapists, dosimetrists, service personnel, and others but given limited reporting authority. This can cause significant problems if personnel are resistant to more time-consuming and complex technologies. As an example, many medical physicists have first-hand experience persuading therapists to perform at the higher level of precision required for stereotactic radiosurgery, IMRT, or 3-D conformal radiotherapy. Secondly, clinic administrators have a significant challenge when asked to manage highly trained and highly compensated professionals such as medical physicists. How can administrators evaluate the performance, productivity, and institutional value of medical physicists unless they have tools by which to measure and evaluate their work? How can medical physicists make persuasive arguments for staffing, space, equipment, and salaries?

The purpose of this chapter is to survey published information that provides a framework for medical physicists and administrators to use in negotiating these resources. Negotiating tactics and philosophy also will be discussed. There is no question that this is a critical topic. As medical physicists, our quality of life, even our livelihood, may well depend on how well we master this information and how convincingly we present the arguments.

2. Determining the framework of the medical physics profession

As we begin the survey, medical physicists must answer some fundamental questions about the profession.

- *Whom do we serve, what do we do for them, and how are we viewed?* Is our client the chief physician, the institutional chief executive officer, the government official, the Medicare representative, the insurance company actuaries, the insurance purchasers for the local major corporations, or the patient?

- *To whom do I report?* Is it the physician, the administrator, the state or Nuclear Regulatory Commission (NRC) inspector, the Joint Commission on Accreditation of Healthcare Organizations (JCAHO) representative, or perhaps another medical physicist for peer review?

- *Who are we, and what do we do?* Is our activity defined by standards of practice, state or federal regulations, task group reports, the JCAHO requirements, or the bylaws of our state's practice act?

- *What is the result if we fail in our responsibilities?* Will I be shunned? Can I be fired? Will I lose my license? Will I go to jail? Will I be sued? Will my institution lose referrals? Will I be removed from the state list of approved consultants? Will my picture appear in the newspaper?

- *What goals do we have in common with managers with respect to the future of our service?* Is it better science with a demonstrable benefit for the patients? Will we have more visibility in the public eye, more appreciation for what we do, and better access to patients? Will we work with supportive physicians and better trained, more enlightened regulatory officials or will the reverse be closer to the mark? How can we increase the probability that we will have enough resources to accomplish these goals? The answers will certainly color and perhaps even determine the outcome of the negotiation process before it begins.

It is not too great a stretch to say that many of the differences medical physicists have result from answering these questions differently, and as a result, making different choices as to where to most strategically focus our efforts. I submit that the patient is in charge and that the medical physicist must always work in the best interest of the patient, even if that means working against the interests of managers or physicians. Whereas the physician may direct the work of the medical physicist, only an appropriate physics peer review can provide the reporting information the manager needs to make critical decisions regarding physics personnel resources. Medical physicists must demonstrate that their practice meets published standards and be willing to suffer the consequences for professional or personal failure. The future is bright, but only if appropriate focus, authority, standards, and accountability lay the foundation for future advancement of the profession.

2.1. The patient's expectations of the medical physicist

Patients who undergo radiological procedures are often unaware of the contributions of medical physicists; however, they are usually aware of some of the problems that require a medical physicist's skill. Most women who read popular magazines know that when they have a mammogram it is important that a good image be obtained without too much radiation exposure. They know that they should look for an accreditation certificate from the American College of Radiology (ACR) as verification that the person performing the scan is qualified. A cancer patient has so many things to worry about, not the least of which is "Am I receiving the proper radiation dose during my radiation treatments?" Many times, patients have legitimate questions about procedures and treatments, but their questions are usually answered by the radiation therapist or physician. Medical physicists are seldom seen or acknowledged by patients, and many medical physicists do little to encourage greater patient interaction.

2.2. The physician's expectations of the medical physicist

Physicians expect medical physicists to implement and manage both routine and special procedures. In addition, they expect the medical physicist to consult with them if a patient presents with an unusual or difficult clinical problem. The medical physicist is expected to maintain quality and to be the technical expert of last resort. Technology has become so complex that it now overwhelms most physicians as well as many radiation therapists. Many physicians view medical physicists as support personnel: technical experts who work under their clinical direction. Not all medical physicists will agree with this assessment, preferring to view medical physics as an independent professional service. Both agree, however, that with respect to clinical matters, the medical physicist should report to the medical director (American College of Radiology 1994).

2.3. The administrator's expectations of the medical physicist

Administrators expect medical physicists to maintain equipment and supervise the imaging, dose-planning, and dose-delivery processes. Medical physicists are expected to maintain the clinical program in top shape for the occasional state, NRC, JCAHO, ACR, or other inspection. Only rarely do managers ask medical physicists to take the lead in community awareness, publicity, or fund-raising projects; however, these marketing functions are vital aspects of operating any business, and medical physicists can increase their perceived value by participating and showing leadership in these areas.

For many managers, the bottom line is the bottom line, and any aspect of the business must justify its value to the business as a whole. With respect to revenue generation, there is a sharp trend toward consolidating and simplifying the patient billing process. Radiation oncology physicists are able to point to a revenue stream to which they contribute; however, the medical-physics-specific codes are under attack. Although diagnostic and nuclear medicine physicists cannot point to specific codes, all radiology services are subject to the wave of cost containment. Medical physics services come at a high price, and it is difficult for medical physicists to avoid being viewed as a cost center. To maintain value in this environment, medical physicists must be able to demonstrate innovation, leadership, and superior performance. Medical physicists are viewed as essential to the operation of the clinic; however, they may be viewed as costly, and their performance may be difficult to evaluate. Given the difficulty of understanding and creating a framework for evaluating a medical physicist's performance, it is important that this task be assigned to upper management. With respect to administrative matters, the medical physicist should be accountable to the appropriate senior administrator, e.g., vice president (American College of Radiology 1994).

3. Establishing the medical physicist's role on the health care team

3.1. The qualified medical physicist

The first definition of a qualified medical physicist was published by the American College of Medical Physics (ACMP) in 1986. In 1993, that definition was revised to include the following summary statement: "The American College of Medical Physics regards board certification, in the appropriate medical physics subfield, and state licensure, in those states in which licensure exists, as the appropriate qualification for the designation of a Qualified Medical Physicist." Similar statements were adopted by the American Association of Physicists in Medicine (AAPM) and the ACR in 1994 and 1996, respectively. Although the definitions differ in some particulars, the common feature is that board certification in the specialty of practice is required to be considered a qualified medical physicist. The significance of the qualified medical physicist from a manager's perspective was explained in an article series by Michael D. Mills, PhD (Mills 1994). If an unqualified physicist is hired to assume final clinic responsibilities, management is exposed to significant liability if anything goes wrong.

3.2. Medical physics practice standards

Very early in the negotiation process, the medical physicist should communicate to the appropriate manager what qualifications are expected or required for a medical physicist to practice independently. If the medical physicist practices in a state that requires a license, he or she may wish to give the administrator selected portions of the state medical physics practice act and associated bylaws.

It also may be helpful to provide the manager with some appropriate brochures or articles to read. Excellent introductions to the field of medical physics have been published by the AAPM, the ACR, the ACMP, and the American Society for Therapeutic Radiology and Oncology (ASTRO). ACR accreditation is mandatory for mammography reimbursement and highly desirable for a radiation oncology program. It is appropriate to introduce the manager to pertinent standards of practice established by the ACR and the ACMP, as these standards are designed to benefit the patient. At times, it also may be advantageous to introduce the manager to selected state radiation regulations, NRC requirements, or JCAHO standards. If new special procedures are considered, the appropriate AAPM task group report may prove helpful. Once again, accurate and verifiable information is key to laying the foundation for a successful negotiation. It is likely many managers will not understand the value of medical physics services unless they appreciate how medical physicists are integrated into the overall health care delivery and regulatory network.

3.3. Professional failure

If the medical physicist fails to perform assigned duties in a professional manner, the consequences are significant. Treatments may be compromised, leading to disease recurrence, injury, or death. The manager faces the loss of patients and revenue, a bad reputation for the department, possible legal actions, disruption of other departments, and possible loss of accreditation or license. The physician faces the loss of patients and revenue, a tarnished reputation in the community, possible legal actions, and a loss of confidence by referring physicians. The physicist faces a loss of reputation, a threat of legal action, possible loss of license or state-approved status, possible employment termination, and even imprisonment. A physicist facing such adversity will certainly need professional counsel and support to negotiate the problem issues. Professional liability issues are addressed by Robert J. Shalek, PhD, in the chapter entitled "The Profession of Medical Physics and Malpractice Issues."

Professional failure by a medical physicist can destroy much more than a single individual. The patients, physicians, managers, and their families all have their lives disrupted, perhaps never to be the same. Medical physicists must take seriously their professional obligation to provide for peer review and practice accreditation. This is especially true as the technology becomes more complex and the special procedures involve greater precision and smaller margin for error.

3.4. Staffing and resource requirements

The potential for program failure illustrates that medical physicists and managers have some common interests with respect to the employment of a medical physicist. In addition to quality, issues such as proper staffing, regulations, practice standards, and overall program success are common and should encourage managers and medical physicists to identify mutual interests and goals regarding employment, resources, and operations within a medical physics program.

Managers require objective and verifiable data on which to base decisions involving resources. There are always places to allocate and spend the revenue, such as advertising, remodeling, and capital equipment. The medical physicist has an obligation to provide published, measured data to support any claim for resources. With respect to staffing, the "Radiation oncology in integrated cancer management" report, the so-called "Blue Book" (Inter-Society Council for Radiation Oncology 1991), is a standard reference that suggests minimum personnel requirements for clinical radiation oncology staffing. Measured staffing profiles for medical physicists, dosimetrists, and other professionals are documented in the report entitled "The Abt study of medical physicist work values for radiation oncology physics services" (American College of Medical Physics 1995). This report breaks out professional staffing profiles based on several categories of practice, including medical school, medical physics consulting, private/community hospital, and medical (physicians) group. Recommendations for staffing levels for diagnostic and nuclear medicine physics services are outlined in a report entitled "Staffing levels and responsibilities of physicists in diagnostic radiology" (American Association of Physicists in Medicine 1997). A similar report was published jointly by the AAPM and the ACMP and was entitled "Recommendations on physics staffing for diagnostic radiology" (American

Institute of Physics 1993). Staffing issues for radiation oncology physics and diagnostic medical physics services are explored further in chapters by Richard G. Lane, PhD ("Medical Physics Staffing Requirements for Radiation Oncology Physics Services") and Stewart C. Bushong, ScD ("Medical Physics Staffing for Diagnostic Imaging").

Radiation oncology special procedures require extensive physics involvement and resources. The ACMP task group report "Survey of physics resources for radiation oncology special procedures" (American College of Medical Physics 1998) measured equipment and personnel start-up resources, ongoing efforts, and costs needed to perform procedures such as total-skin electron irradiation, electron arc therapy, high-dose-rate brachytherapy, stereotactic brachytherapy, intraoperative radiotherapy, total-body irradiation, stereotactic radiosurgery, and 3-D treatment planning. Procedure costs, including personnel time and equipment, were measured through a survey and subsequent data analysis of information provided by the 109 medical physicists responding. This document provides the administrator with the information required to plan and budget resources to tackle new programs with confidence.

Salary survey information is published each year by the AAPM. It is usually possible to persuade administrators that new hires should be employed at the 50% to 80% salary range. This will allow the clinic to recruit personnel of sufficient quality while maintaining a range for merit increases.

4. The negotiation process

Up to this point, we have discussed the framework and the resources the medical physicist will need for negotiation. Now we must address the question of how the negotiation should proceed. Medical physicists are usually at a disadvantage when they negotiate with administrators. This is true even when medical physicists are prepared with the facts and documentation to support their case. Principals of negotiation are usually not part of the training and education of a medical physicist, whereas administrators consider negotiating an essential tool for business success. Some excellent resource materials have come from Harvard's Program on Negotiation and have been documented in popular books by Robert Fisher and William Ury (Fisher and Ury 1981; Ury 1993). Frequently, administrators attend seminars and workshops to sharpen negotiating skills. With the growth of teams, a structure in which there is no clear authority, negotiating skills are especially critical. Successful negotiation involves meticulous preparation, understanding both side's needs, and an ability to build rapport and trust. If there is an ongoing relationship involved, success is making both sides feel good about the outcome.

The most difficult and essential part of negotiating is listening to the other side. Communication is key. You may wish to restate your opponent's position in your own words until they are satisfied that you understand. Instead of being their problem, try to become part of the team trying to solve their problem. Instead of attacking one another, jointly attack the problem. Recognize that joint problem solving revolves around interests instead of positions.

It helps for a medical physicist to understand and list his or her own professional interests as well as those of the opponent in order to understand how interests determine a negotiating position. For example, the medical physicist's interests might be to: 1) continue to provide the highest-quality radiation treatment by generating standards for radiation oncology operation processes, negotiating agreement and support for those standards, and requiring adherence to those standards; 2) continue to grow professionally and to develop experience administrating an intermediate-size physics program with line management authority for that program; 3) provide new services such as 3-D treatment planning, IMRT, and prostate brachytherapy treatments as part of radiation oncology practice over the next 3 to 5 years; and 4) be in the top 10% of our profession with respect to level of responsibility, job performance, and compensation.

An administrator's interests might be to: 1) operate a clinic in a manner that demonstrates shrewd management through operational and financial achievement; 2) spend as little as possible on clinic salaries (usually no more than 30% of total clinic revenue is devoted to salaries); 3) save money by providing emerging technology only when such technology is required by market conditions such as competition from another clinic or demands from referring physicians; 4) hire the best people available at no more than the median salary for the position, allowing room for merit awards and salary advancements; 5) cap the highest level of salary for a position at the 80th percentile of the survey; and 6) limit the authority of highly paid professionals in favor of a teamwork approach.

Barriers to cooperation with administration might include your angry reaction to their position; their emotional response if you disagree or reject their offer; their position when it is offered as non-negotiable; their dissatisfaction if the proposed agreement does not take into account their interests; and their power if it is used to force compliance while destroying the relationship with the medical physicist. Remember, victory is making both sides feel satisfied. There are wise and proper reactions to these barriers.

- Your angry reaction to their position: Imagine yourself standing on a balcony looking down on your negotiation. Control your anger. Think as though you were a disinterested advisor to the proceedings.

- Their emotional response if you disagree or reject their offer: Step to their side, listen to them, acknowledge their points and their feelings, agree with them, and show them respect. Repeat their positions and interests until they are satisfied that you understand. Take a coffee break.

- Their position when offered as non-negotiable: Take their position and probe it. Act as though they are your partners on a team that is out to find a solution to the problem. Test every assumption between their interests and their position. Look for a creative alternative proposal.

- Their dissatisfaction if the proposed agreement does not take into account their interests: Bridge the gap between their interests and yours. Help them to save face, and make the outcome look like a victory for them. Look for ways to preserve and build the relationship.

- Their power: Show them they cannot win by themselves, only together with you. Work to remind them that victory and the preservation of the relationship is only possible when both sides feel satisfied with the outcome.

Before every meeting, prepare; after every meeting, assess your progress, adapt your strategy, and prepare again. Be patient, medical physicists are often consumed with the desire to solve the problem as soon as possible. Recognize that negotiation is a journey, and there are specific signposts that indicate progress is being made. There are five important points along the way to a mutually satisfactory agreement: identifying interests, identifying options for satisfying those interests, setting standards for resolving differences fairly, choosing alternatives to negotiation, and proposing an agreement.

- Identifying interests: Interests are not dollars, terms, and conditions but rather intangible motivations that lead you to take a position—your needs, concerns, fears, and aspirations. (Refer to the list of interests above.)

- Identifying options for satisfying those interests: An option is a possible agreement or part of an agreement. Options usually generate different responses among opponents; however, options are useful, because they expose perspectives and expectations with respect for how the problem may be resolved.

- Setting standards for resolving differences: A standard is a measuring stick that allows you to decide what is a fair solution. If you and your opponent agree on standards, an important milestone has been reached.

- Choosing alternatives to negotiate: Knowing what your alternatives are can determine your success in satisfying your interests. Your BATNA—best alternative to a negotiated agreement (keep it secret)—is your best course of action for satisfying your interests without the other party's agreement. If you can identify the other party's BATNA, you will know the limit of what you can achieve in the negotiation. Even so, an agreement just short of your opponent's BATNA may not allow him or her to save face. Remember that a successful agreement also meets the needs of your opponent.

- Proposing an agreement: Before going into your final negotiating session, divide possible proposals to which you are ready to say yes into three categories:

What do I aspire to? What would I be content with? What could I live with? Have the answers to these questions written down before you negotiate. Do not accept an alternative that does not meet your minimum criteria; instead, postpone the agreement until you have a chance to think about the proposal at your leisure.

Tactics that may be used by your opponent to gain the upper hand include: 1) stone wall, a refusal to budge from a position; 2) attacks, a pressure tactic designed to intimidate you and make you feel so uncomfortable that you give in to the other side's demands; and 3) tricks, tactics that dupe you into giving in. Handling the tactics involves patience. Pause and say nothing. Be quick to hear, slow to speak, and slow to act. Rewind the tape; replay the conversation first in your mind and then out loud. Review the negotiation and discussion to this point. Take a time-out and have a coffee break. Do not let yourself be hurried. Only you can make the concession you will later regret. Step to their side; listen to what they have to say; acknowledge their point, their feelings, and their competence and status; and agree with them wherever you can. When tempted to anger, remember these words:

> "Speak when you are angry and you will make
> the best speech you will ever regret."
> --*Ambrose Bierce*

5. Conclusion

The pressures of managed care place an enormous strain on the delicate process of negotiation between health care administrators and health care workers. A medical physicist must think carefully about the profession and reflect on his or her role on the health care team. Educating the administrator about the structure and function of medical physics in the health care environment is an essential first step in negotiating. The negotiation process depends on the ability to identify a solution that meets their mutual needs and interests and preserves the relationship. The medical physicist should prepare for this process as if it were the most important test ever faced. It is important to anticipate tactics used by the opponent to control the process. Do not respond to unexpected tactics, and do not allow the opponent to hurry the process.

Negotiating with administrators requires perspective, preparation, patience, and perseverance. At bottom, satisfaction with your employment depends largely on what you are able to negotiate. Frustration with your situation often results from not having the confidence that you can continue to negotiate the best situation for yourself. The information gleaned in this chapter is a first step toward developing a lifestyle in which successful negotiation leads to peace of mind that you have done your best for yourself and your family.

References

Abt Associates Inc. (1995) "The Abt study of medical physicists work values for radiation oncology physics services." Cambridge, MA:Abt Associates Inc.

American Association of Physicists in Medicine (1991) "Staffing levels and responsibilities of physicists in diagnostic radiology," AAPM Report No. 33. Woodbury, NY:AIP

— (1997) "Professional information survey report—Calendar year 1996," AAPM Professional Survey Subcommittee, Professional Information and Clinical Relations Committee, and Professional Council Report. College Park, MD: AAPM

American College of Medical Physics (1998) "Survey of physics resources for radiation oncology special procedures," ACMP Task Group Report. Reston, VA: ACMP

American College of Radiology (1994) "ACR standard for radiation oncology physics for external beam therapy," ACR Commission on Standards and Accreditation. Reston, VA:ACR

American Institute of Physics (1993) "Recommendations on physics staffing for diagnostic radiology," A report of the Trilateral Committee of the AAPM, ACMP, and ACR Commission on Physics. Woodbury, NY:AIP

Fisher R and Ury W (1981) Getting to yes. Boston, MA:Houghton Mifflin

Inter-Society Council for Radiation Oncology (1991) "Radiation oncology in integrated cancer management." Philadelphia, PA:ACR

Mills MD (1994) Implications of licensure of medical physicists: A study in risk management and quality improvement, Parts 1 and 2. *Administrative Radiology* **13**(2),45-51 and **13**(3),41-45

Ury W (1993) Getting past no. New York, NY:Bantam

Michael D. Mills, PhD

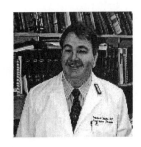

Michael D. Mills received his PhD in Biomedical Science with emphasis on radiation biology at The University of Texas Graduate School of Biomedical Sciences in Houston, TX in 1980. Dr. Mills subsequently received postdoctoral training in therapeutic radiological physics in the Department of Physics at The University of Texas M. D. Anderson Hospital and Tumor Institute (now The University of Texas M. D. Anderson Cancer Center) in Houston, TX in 1981. He then worked from 1981 to 1983 as a staff physicist at Cleveland Clinic in Cleveland, OH and from 1983 to 1988 as an Assistant Professor in the Department of Radiation Physics at M. D. Anderson Cancer Center. From 1988 to1998, Dr. Mills was a consulting physicist in his own company, Misslou Medical Physics, serving small to medium-size cancer centers in Mississippi and Louisiana. He is presently directing physics and dosimetry at the University of Louisville Brown Cancer Center in Louisville, KY. Dr. Mills has been very active in the major professional organizations of medical physicists, having chaired and served on numerous committees. He is presently the ACMP representative to the JCAHO and Chairman of the ACMP Commission on Professional Practice. He led the ACMP-AAPM project "The Abt study of medical physicists work values for radiation oncology physics services." He also was a major contributor to the ACMP study "Survey of physics resources for radiation oncology special procedures." Dr. Mills is a Fellow of the ACMP and is well known for his interest in and contributions to medical physics professional issues.

Professional Interactions with Physicians and with Allied Health Professionals

Michael T. Gillin, PhD

Department of Radiation Oncology, Medical College of Wisconsin, Milwaukee, WI

Abstract. Professional interactions with oncologists and other staff in the allied health field are important in the practice of medical physics. This interaction should be based on the ethical, religious, and philosophical values that form the foundation of our lives and our civilization. Interactions between physicists and oncologists can be particularly challenging because of their cultural differences, and sustained effort is required to ensure that these professionals interact effectively. This work presents my experience and insight in addressing common challenges that occur when physicists interact with oncologists, other physicists, therapists, and other medical professionals. Specific situations, such as dealing with dosimetric errors, are presented. As a physicist, I have learned that if I hold myself to the highest personal and professional standards, then my colleagues will, for the most part, interact with me at that level.

1. Introduction

Disclaimers are appropriate when creating a work such as this. As a medical physicist, I have no specific training in the area of human interactions. In fact, people close to me might suggest that as a Newtonian-thinking physicist, I have some handicaps in this complex area. The information presented here reflects over 25 years of experience as a medical physicist, and I believe that professional relationships have represented the largest challenge of my career.

In 1974, at the age of 33, I was planning on resigning from the Army and looking for my first nonmilitary job. I asked for advice from Robert J. Shalek, PhD, who is now professor emeritus at The University of Texas M. D. Anderson Cancer Center, Houston, TX. Dr. Shalek advised me to associate myself with radiation oncologists who were good physicians and who were decent human beings and not to be too concerned about the other details. His wisdom remains appropriate today.

My professional career has been spent at two different locations. The first 4 years were spent at Walter Reed Army Medical Center, where I had the privilege of being associated with a wise, experienced medical physicist, Bob Quillin, MS, and many fine young radiation oncologists. One of the first principles that Bob taught me was that the oncologist was always in charge. Thus, I understood that medical departments are dictatorships and, for the lucky, the dictator is benign.

For the last 22 years, I have worked at the Medical College of Wisconsin with a group of radiation oncologists whose focus has been and remains quality patient care, medical education, and clinical research. As a faculty member, I am an employee of the school and a member of the group practice. The department chairman is my boss. I have been the senior radiation oncology physicist at this practice since my first day here. It has always been a surprise to me to find myself part of management. I was trained as a physicist, and as such, I enjoy making measurements, testing the limits of computer programs, and even repairing accelerators. I have no formal training in any management area; yet, I supervise at least nine people. Common sense has served me well when I have dealt with situations in which I have not been formally trained. When I lose my grasp of common sense, I seek help from my colleagues and family. As a professional, I am legally required to act in a reasonably prudent manner.

In preparation for this paper, I relied on several resources. One was *The Dilbert Principle* (Adams 1996). The Dilbert Principle evolved from the older Peter Principle, which stated that workers were promoted until they reached their level of incompetence. The Dilbert Principle states that the most ineffective workers are systematically moved to the place where they can do the least damage: management. As a senior medical physicist, I may be an example of the Peter Principle, but I attempt to avoid the errors so humorously described in *The Dilbert Principle* and in the daily comic strip that features the same character. At times in the clinical setting, I have seen the Dilbert Principle in action.

A more serious reference is *The 7 Habits of Highly Effective People* by Stephen R. Covey (Covey 1989). This author correctly points out that the maturity continuum starts at dependence, goes through independence, and ends with interdependence. His seven habits are divided into three private habits (proactive, begin with the end in mind, and put first things first), three public habits, (think win/win, seek first to understand then to be understood, and synergize), and the habit of balanced self-renewal. I believe that medical physicists should strive to be highly effective people.

Another reference that I find quite interesting is *Love and Profit, The Art of Caring Leadership* by James A. Autry (Autry 1991). This author discusses work as a community, a new neighborhood. I have come to view my department of radiation oncology as my community, as I spend a substantial amount of time there. Autry states that work should provide the opportunity for spiritual and personal growth and notes that we are wasting too much time at work if it fails to do so. I believe that there are spiritual and personal growth opportunities in serving patients through the practice of medical physics. Autry also notes that good management is largely a matter of caring for people.

There are textbooks for students on management that focus on a variety of related topics, such as organizational behavior and human relationships. Issues addressed in such works include communication, motivation, leadership, and conflict resolution. There are many other references at the local bookstore that address issues related to professional interactions. In my opinion, it is important for medical physicists to become familiar with some of these works, because professionally, we interact with people from a wide spectrum of backgrounds.

2. Basic principles of professional interaction

Our parents were correct. The principles of life that we were all taught as children are the basis upon which all human relationships are built. These principles include the Golden Rule and characteristics such as integrity, fidelity, justice, patience, and industry. Covey describes this in his discussion of the character ethic. I believe that there are natural laws, some of which are expressed as ethical, religious, and moral principles, that should govern all of our behavior.

Our parents also reminded us that we are responsible for our own actions. This turns out to be a principle in law. Medical physicists have unique responsibilities and are responsible for their own actions, whether they be actions of commission or omission. The same is true for all professionals.

Polite behavior is always expected, just as our parents insisted. It is my opinion that professional relationships are always to be conducted in a polite fashion. The more intense the situation, the greater the need for politeness. Sometimes it is very difficult to discipline oneself to be polite. However, in my personal experience, I have always regretted my lapses from this standard. Even if you are disagreeing, disagree politely.

2.1. Interactions with the department chairperson

The department chairperson is the boss, even if the physicist does not report directly to the person in this position. Generally, the department chairperson works very closely with the highest-level administrators in the institution. Physicists need the support of the chairperson. Negotiations with the chairperson regarding physics concerns must be conducted in a polite, respectful manner. From the perspective of the physicist, there may never be sufficient resources to meet all of the physics responsibilities. From the perspective of the chairman, every section of the department is demanding more resources. Reasonable negotiations between reasonable people do not always result in everyone being satisfied. It is important for the medical physicist to understand this and to consider the options. For some time, my chairman and I have agreed to disagree on a number of issues. If the situation is one in which, because of limited resources or increased responsibility, I believed that standards of practice are not being met and if after long discussions with the chairman there is no resolution, then it is my opinion that one of the few honorable options left open to me would be to seek other employment. It is interesting to note that the standards of practice for radiation oncology physics have been and are continuously being defined in documents such as the American Association of Physicists in Medicine (AAPM) task group reports (American Association of Physicists in Medicine 1993, 1994a, 1994b, and 1995) and the American College of Medical Physics (ACMP) and American College of Radiology (ACR) standards (American College of Medical Physics 1986; American College of Radiology 1996a, 1996b, 1996c). These documents are helpful in evaluating specific situations; however, there is a point at which it is not possible to defend the failure to perform certain actions, and the physicist has no choice but to resign. Even under such dire circumstances, the interaction between the chairman and the physicist must be conducted in the most polite, respectful manner possible.

2.2. Interactions with staff radiation oncologists

In theory, the relationship between the radiation oncologist and the medical physicist should be simple. The oncologist provides clinical services and the physicist provides physics services. My relationships with oncologists, however, have been complex for several reasons. Each oncologist wants something slightly different in the way of physics support. At times there is tension, because the oncologist wants his or her request given the highest priority. It has been my experience that it is difficult to keep a group of eight radiation oncologists satisfied at all times with the physics services they receive. For example, questions arise as to why time is being spent on prostate implants rather than on stereotactic radiosurgery. In such a circumstance, I attempt to communicate the tasks to be performed and the resources available to perform these tasks. In my opinion, it is reasonable for me to educate the oncologists relative to specific physics issues and to review departmental priorities. At times, departmental priorities and expectations are not consistent with departmental resources.

Physicists provide unique services to oncologists, such as the calibration of the radiation sources. The oncologist must trust that the physicist has met his or her responsibilities in an appropriate manner. This trust is something that the medical physicist must earn and constantly maintain. It is maintained through interactions that are conducted in an honest, intelligent, respectful, and polite manner. If the physicist is uncertain about a specific source calibration, the physicist needs to communicate that uncertainty to the oncologist. Examples of such source calibration uncertainties might include the calibration of a superficial or contact unit or of a Sr-90 eye applicator. It is prudent to first communicate this uncertainty verbally and then to communicate it in a written format. It is unreasonable for oncologists to assume that every physicist has the training, experience, and equipment to provide accurate calibrations of all radiation sources available in a large clinic. It is reasonable for the physicist to request help from a consultant or colleague to ensure that the calibration is properly performed, thus ensuring that the element of trust remains.

As a consultant, I have been to clinics where the oncologists no longer trusted the physicists. The causes of the lack of trust ranged from specific incidents in which the oncologist felt that the physicist did not display sufficient integrity to general complaints about lack of physics effort. It has been my experience that there is no way for the physicist to salvage this situation, and the physicist is best advised to seek employment elsewhere. Once the physician staff loses trust in the physicist, it is impossible to replace. The opposite is also true. If the physicist looses trust or confidence in the actions and judgments of the oncologists, it is time to seek other employment.

Radiation oncologists and medical physicists come from two different cultures, because they represent two different educational and training processes. Physicians have memorized large amounts of material that represents the clinical experience of other physicians, and they base many of their clinical decisions on this material. Physicists have been trained to start from fundamentals and apply them to the problem at hand. These differences in culture are important to remember as they have an impact on how we interact with each other. I feel that one of the most valuable lessons that years of experience have taught me is the understanding of the thought processes used by the radiation oncologists to solve specific problems. As a physicist, I must know basic radiation oncology, such as the goals of a specific treatment, the basic departmental treatment approaches, and the specific concerns unique to individual oncologists. Understanding on my part will lead to a more effective interaction. The oncologists expect the medical physicist to have a basic understanding of clinical situations, and medical physicists expect oncologists to have a basic understanding of physics and dosimetry. Senior medical physicists should be able to recognize the unsolvable dosimetric problem and to discuss this with the oncologists. For example, a dose gradient of less than 10% through a tangential breast field is simply not possible for certain patient contours. This should be recognized and discussed with the oncologist. The treatment planner's time can then be redirected toward solvable problems.

I am routinely summoned to the clinic to provide a physics consultation regarding a specific patient. It is my general impression that I have approximately 30 seconds to produce an intelligent statement, because the oncologists have many demands on their time. Many consultations are routine, such as discussing the merits of electron versus orthovoltage treatments. Sometimes, however, the most intelligent thing I have said is that I do not know the answer to the question at hand. One example of this is when an oncologist once asked me why a treatment unit was causing a specific reaction (or lack thereof) in a patient. It is my opinion that radiation oncologists appreciate and respect the honest statement of ignorance, with an offer to pursue the appropriate answer. I attempt to avoid the intelligent guess.

Interacting with the noninterested oncologist can be a challenge. Recently, while discussing the dosimetric aspects of a four-field breast treatment, the staff oncologist informed me that he was not interested in all the details. I felt insulted and angry. In this case, I documented the details of that patient's treatment in the same manner as I would any other four-field breast patient. My goal was to meet my responsibility to the patient and to the oncologist, even if the oncologist exhibited limited interest. It is my opinion that I had acted in a consistent and prudent fashion. I had not embarrassed the oncologist by either not writing appropriate documentation in the chart or by writing nonprofessional comments, although I must confess that I was tempted to do so.

The rule in my department is that as the senior person in physics and dosimetry, all technical errors are my responsibility. When an error is discovered or suspected, my first action is to verbally inform the staff oncologist and to take full responsibility.

This is done either alone or with others, if others wish to be involved. Together, we discuss what has happened. If need be, the staff oncologist and I will inform the chairman together. The chairman is informed before Risk Management is contacted. It is my position that I should be as honest and as thorough as possible when dealing with dosimetric errors. The first priority is to protect the patient, and the next is to protect the institution. Other issues are secondary. It is my understanding that this "no excuse" approach elevates physics services in the eyes of the oncologist.

2.3. Interactions with medical physicists

Professional relationships between medical physicists working in the same group require mutual patience and respect. At times, I find this to be a challenge. I am sure that all of us feel that in certain instances we could have performed the task better or faster or with greater precision. However, with the exception of incompetence, the task has been performed in an adequate manner. My own work style is to work alone and then to provide a report to my physics colleagues on the task. Others prefer to work in groups. There are multiple approaches to any task, and we must respect and be patient with whatever approach is used.

Professional relationships between medical physicists require good communication. In theory, because of the similar training of physicists, communication between physicists should be easy. It is my general experience that this is true. One result of this communication is the independent review of the work product of physicists by physics colleagues, protecting both the patient and the physicist. Independent physics review should generally be performed before the project is discussed with the oncologist. One benefit of good communication between physicists is a unity in the physics position. It is common, in my experience, for several physicists to be asked the same clinical or administrative question by the same individual. When our answers are different, it usually causes confusion or problems. Our regularly scheduled, weekly physics/dosimetry conference has aided communication in my practice.

Fortunately, it has been decades since I worked alone. I am not sure that I could function as a single physicist at an institution, because I am most comfortable when interacting with my physics colleagues. If placed in the position of working alone, I would attempt to obtain funds for consultants and to establish a collegial relationship with a physicist at a noncompetitive institution for the purpose of providing each other with peer review.

2.4. Interactions with individuals supervised by the medical physicist

The Golden Rule of "treating others as you wish to be treated" is an excellent approach to take in professional interactions with those you supervise. One characteristic that I have attempted to display as a manager is to be a good listener. When dosimetrists, engineers, or block makers come to me to discuss a topic, I attempt to listen carefully and think creatively. I certainly appreciate this characteristic in those from whom I have sought advise. One habit that is worth learning well is to express appreciation for a task well performed. We all enjoy being told that we have done a good job. The individuals we supervise also enjoy this. I like to write letters of commendation praising an individual for a task well done. This also helps me for annual evaluations.

The Golden Rule is not enough, however. The difficult employee is a challenge for us all. In fact, managing the difficult employee may be the worst part of any manager's job, and it is certainly the worst part of my job. My advice is to seek help from others, such as your Human Resources Department, and to keep your superiors well informed.

2.5. Interactions with individuals not supervised by the medical physicist

A good working relationship between therapists and physicists is very important. At times, therapists are the first group to experience machine problems. One basic rule in our clinic is that when the therapist requests our help or informs us of a problem, we should listen, attempt to address the issue, and report back to the therapist, even if it is a negative report. In addition, we should discuss the issue with the therapist's supervisor. This results in a win/win situation. I believe that the physicist must provide almost instantaneous support to the therapist to ensure safe and appropriate treatment delivery to the patient.

As treatments become more complex, the therapist and the physicist should be working together more closely. A written acknowledgment from the physicist to the departmental director when a therapist has performed in a commendable manner is appreciated by everyone. Conversely, if there is a problem with the therapist, it is prudent for the physicist to discuss this problem with both the therapist and the director. A bad working relationship between the therapist and the physicist will make the physicist's activities more difficult and will increase the risks to the patients. It has been my experience that patience, respect, and time have permitted my relationships with some therapists to mature into effective working partnerships.

Every physicist who receives any clerical support should be appreciative of that support. I attempt to have realistic expectations of clerical support, especially because the individual providing that support also is supporting others. When I have a big project coming up, I discuss this project with those who will be providing me with support. It is my responsibility to be aware of deadlines and to complete my work within a reasonable lead time.

3. Summary

As a physicist in medicine, I believe that I am the one on the health care team who is from a different culture. After more then 25 years, I am still discovering cultural differences that distinguish me from my clinical colleagues. As the visitor in this foreign culture, I need to be at my best. Communication between members from different cultures requires sustained effort. To the oncologists and others, I need to communicate physics in as accurate and succinct a manner as possible. In the foreign culture of medicine, it is wise for me to acknowledge my limitations and to request help. Sometimes I need to communicate in the foreign languages of medicine and business. In this area, I need to be especially concerned about the accuracy of my communications. However, I do want to communicate in these languages, as I feel I have important contributions to make, and actions in these areas will affect me.

In my practice as a radiation oncology physicist, I am aware of the fact that I am being evaluated through my verbal and written communications and through my actions. Thus, I should communicate to the oncologists and others my successes, such as an independent review that indicates that the accelerator has been appropriately calibrated. I should communicate my major activities, such as the calibration, operation, and repair history of major treatment devices during the past year, as is recommended by AAPM Task Group Report 40 (American Association of Physicists in Medicine 1994a) and by the ACR "Standard for radiation oncology physics for external beam therapy" (American College of Radiology 1996a). I should communicate major advances in my areas of interest, such as the impact of AAPM Task Group Report 43 on I-125 dose calculations (American Association of Physicists in Medicine 1995). For new procedures, I should communicate my needs for training and equipment as is recommended in the ACR "Standard for radiation oncology physics for external beam therapy" (American College of Radiology 1996a). I also should communicate my concerns, as I have unique responsibilities to the patients who seek care at my facility as is discussed in AAPM Task Group Report 35 (American Association of Physicists in Medicine 1993).

It has been my good fortune to be associated, for the most part, with intelligent, caring colleagues, including oncologists, physicists, dosimetrists, therapists, and others. I feel a strong responsibility to work interdependently with them in providing quality care. I need to interact in the most professional manner possible, and I expect my colleagues to also meet this high standard. Professional relationships constitute an important element in my life.

References

Adams S (1996) The Dilbert Principle. New York: Harper Business

American Association of Physicists in Medicine (1993) "Medical accelerator safety considerations," Report of AAPM Radiation Therapy Committee Task Group 35. *Medical Physics* **20**,1261-1275

— (1994a) "Comprehensive QA for radiation oncology," Report of AAPM Radiation Therapy Committee Task Group 40. *Medical Physics* **21**,581-618

— (1994b) "Code of practice for radiotherapy accelerators," Report of AAPM Radiation Therapy Committee Task Group 45. *Medical Physics* **21**,1093-1124

— (1995) "Dosimetry of interstitial brachytherapy sources," Report of AAPM Radiation Therapy Committee Task Group 43. *Medical Physics* **22**,209-234

American College of Medical Physics (1986) "Radiation control and quality assurance in radiation oncology: A suggestion protocol," ACMP Report No. 2. Reston, VA:ACMP

American College of Radiology (1996a) "Standard for radiation oncology physics for external beam therapy," ACR Standard. Reston, VA:ACR

— (1996b) "Standard for the performance of brachytherapy physics:Manually loaded sources," ACR Standard. Reston, VA:ACR

— (1996c) "Standard for the performance of high-dose-rate brachytherapy," ACR Standard. Reston, VA: ACR

Autry JA (1991) Love and Profit. The Art of Caring Leadership. New York, NY:Avon Books

Covey SR (1989) The 7 Habits of Highly Effective People. New York, NY:Fireside

Michael T. Gillin, PhD

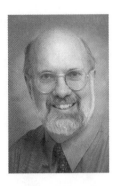

Michael T. Gillin received his PhD in Physics from the University of California, Davis in 1970. Afterwards, as part of his 5 years of service in the U.S. Army's Medical Service Corps, he did a Radiological Physics Fellowship at the Walter Reed Army Medical Center. In 1975, Dr. Gillin joined the faculty at the Medical College of Wisconsin, where he is now Professor and Chief Physicist in the Department of Radiation Oncology. He is well known for his research contributions in brachytherapy and quality assurance. Dr. Gillin is active in numerous professional and scientific societies. He has been Chairman of the ACMP, Parliamentarian of the AAPM, and has served on numerous committees of the ACR. He is a Fellow of the ACMP and an Honorary Certified Medical Dosimetrist. Dr. Gillin has been very active in the Radiation Therapy Oncology Group, having served as Chairman of the Physics Committee from 1990 to 1997. His interactions with a variety of health care professionals in radiation oncology make him a selection well suited for this topic.

Financial Issues

Billing for Physics Procedures

Ann E. Wright, PhD

Ann E. Wright, PhD and Associates, Houston, TX

Abstract. To understand the complexities of billing for physics services rendered to patients, one must review the 20th century evolution of health care in the United States. The introduction of technologically advanced medical devices utilizing electronics, computers, and high-energy radiation required full-time participation of the medically trained physicist. Methods of financing nonphysician professionals had to be created and fitted into the reimbursement schemes extant in the early 1970s. Because provision and reimbursement of patient services by hospitals and physicians has undergone a revolution from private fee-for-service practice, through government provision of health care to the elderly, to the health management organizations of today, reimbursement for the medical physicist's services is now at risk. The protection afforded the medical physicist's position in the past by physician colleagues is threatened by the drive toward cost containment in medical care. Although great strides have been made in the certification area, the need for licensure and special legislation for the medical physicist is greater than ever.

1. Introduction

Billing for physics procedures might appear to be a simple and prosaic subject, with a moderate level of complexity. On the contrary, it is a many-sided and complex matter, with the elements constantly changing. To grasp the topic, one must review not only the past, present, and future of billing and reimbursement for physics procedures, but also the origin and development of medical physics as an occupation.

The application of modern physics to the medical area is a phenomenon of the 20th century. Medical physics, as an occupation, grew from the development of technologically advanced medical equipment requiring the services of a university-trained physicist both in medical education and patient-care areas. In the beginning, both industry and medicine looked to the physics faculty at nearby universities for scientific input. In the early days, the excitement of research with exotic instruments and the intangible reward of helping the less fortunate led faculty members to donate considerable time and effort. As demands on their time grew beyond what could be reasonably accommodated, sources of funding for full-time physicists on medical school faculties were sought.

As the use of complex radiological equipment expanded into community hospitals, manpower needs grew, leading to the establishment of medical physics training programs. It was thought necessary to incorporate courses in biology, physiology, and anatomy in order to facilitate communication between the physician and the physicist. The medical physicist became not only a teacher but a consultant to the physician regarding the design and application of radiation for diagnosis and treatment. In recognition of the medical physicist's contribution, mechanisms were established to reimburse those services similar to the reimbursement for the physician's services in patient care.

Although the occupation of medical physics has existed for only a relatively few years (about 4 decades) many changes in society and in the health care area have shaped both its scientific and professional development. In this chapter, I will present highlights from this era. For those who want more detail about the role the federal government plays in providing health care for the elderly, an overview of the Medicare program is presented in an appendix to this chapter.

2. Historical development of the medical physics profession

2.1. Highlights of the 1960s

The decade of the 1960s was a period of unprecedented demand for new cars, homes, appliances, and consumer goods leading to a booming economy. Increased profits for business and manufacturers led to increased research budgets and advances in technology. New technologies found their way into doctors' offices and hospitals. Physicists and engineers involved in developing new technology were invited to help adapt these technologies for use in patient care. The most seminal of these adaptations for the physicist, of course, was the use of x-rays in diagnostic and treatment applications.

The federal government's initial role in health care was to limit the spread of communicable diseases. This role was expanded during both world wars to include battlefield and hospital patient care. During the 1960s, the National Institutes of Health were broadened to encompass acute disease research. Grants were established to develop new medical equipment and to provide special training for those responsible for the use and maintenance of this equipment. Graduating physics students were recruited to new, degree-offering training programs funded by the National Cancer Institute. Part of the requirement was completion of courses in biology and anatomy and completion of research projects related to medicine. Biomedical science was teamed with electronics, computer science, and materials science to create a revolution in health care and to place greater demands on the physicians.

2.2. Highlights of the 1970s

During the 1970s, the possibility of miracle cures for life-threatening diseases was voiced. A society freed from drudgery and leading increasingly more comfortable lives began to look to the health care industry for relief from the pain of acute and chronic illnesses. Training of physicians became vastly more complex as the "art" of healing gave way to the "science" of healing. The traditional training of the physician had to be expanded to include lessons in the theory and operation of "high tech" equipment; the scientifically trained medical physicist was drafted for this job. The job of designing and executing tests to ensure the safety and reliability of the equipment also was delegated to the medical physicist. Developing computer programs to assist in treatment planning and determining the appropriate equipment for patient care was made safer and more precise by the presence of the medical physicist.

The demand for graduates from the training programs grew as the use of technologically advanced equipment spread to community hospitals. Physicians trained in the use of the equipment negotiated to acquire new technology and hire medical physicists at private or community hospitals. Because there were no faculty salaries for physicists recruited to such hospitals, funds for employment of physicists had to be found. The problem was most acute for medical physicists working in the therapy area and involved in treatment planning for specific patients. The responsibility for the accuracy of both radiation-dose computations and delivery of radiation by the equipment required expenditure of more time than the normal workday encompassed. Because these services fell outside the realm of responsibility of traditional nonphysician health care positions, such as nurses and medical technicians, inappropriate guidelines were often used to assess physics manpower needs. In the absence of budgetary help from other sources, the medical physicists responsible for staffing and equipping a medical physics department had to become resourceful.

The need for funding for the clinical physicist in the early 1970s led to parallel efforts on the part of physicists in several areas of the country. A group of medical physicists in Texas approached the Blue Cross and Blue Shield of Texas, Inc. (the insurance carrier contracted to handle Medicare as well as a large number of private patients) requesting acceptance and payment of medical physicists' charges for services rendered to patients receiving radiation treatment. The following is an excerpt from the letter addressing this issue.

> *Medical Director*
> *Blue Cross and Blue Shield of Texas, Inc.*
> *Dallas, Texas*
>
> *Dear Sir:*
>
> *We feel there are certain areas (of radiotherapy) which should be carried out under the supervision of a medical physicist. (Our) suggestion is to define an adjunctive radiotherapy physics service... necessary to the conduct of radiation therapy for optimal patient care, performed in consultation with a qualified radiological... physicist....(a list of patient services followed including treatment planning, dosimetry, and design and construction of beam-shaping devices.)*

We propose an additional item: Continuing radiological physics services in support of the radiotherapist in patient management (e.g., calibrations, review of dosimetry records, radiation safety), per patient course...

We would like to urge that these listings be included in the codes for Texas.

Subsequent meetings with the medical director led to the recognition and reimbursement of a list of radiotherapy physics charges. Because medical physicists were not licensed in the state at the time and had no standing in law, the charges were classified by Medicare as "services incidental to the services of a physician," and direct billing of the patient by the medical physicist was disallowed. By default, codes for patient services rendered by medical physicists were adopted into the physician (professional) codes and hospital (technical) codes.

The practice arrangements of medical physicists vary, but most fall into one of the following categories: 1) hospital employee; 2) medical school faculty member, with or without salary augmentation from clinical service in a teaching hospital; 3) employee of a physician practice group; 4) member of a medical physicist practice group; 5) employee of a physician-directed clinic or freestanding center; or 6) employee of a government hospital.

Depending on who bears the cost of providing physics services, reimbursement for services rendered to a Medicare patient is made by an "intermediary" to a hospital or through a "carrier" to a physician, a physician group, or a freestanding center. Reimbursement for services rendered to a beneficiary of a private insurance company is made directly by the company to the health care provider (hospital) or to the physician. For additional details about the Medicare system, see Appendix A - The Role of the Health Care Financing Administration.

2.3. Highlights of the 1980s

During the decade of the 1980s, the number of physicists working in the clinical area grew rapidly. In 1974, the American Association of Physicists in Medicine (AAPM) placement service advertised a total of 49 job openings for medical physicists. By 1980, this number had grown to 195, and by the end of 1989, the AAPM listed over 300 job openings per year. In the same period, starting salaries for master's degreed medical physicists grew from around $20,000 per year to $40,000 and above. This salary range attracted some individuals with only minimal qualifications; therefore, certification processes were put in place to measure competence. The American College of Medical Physics (ACMP) published a definition of a "qualified medical physicist," which was written into the regulatory requirements in several states.

On the economic front, double-digit inflation led to a public outcry for the government to lower taxes and government expenditures. With health care expenditures growing at the rate of about 15% per year, hospitals and physicians became targets for politicians and bureaucrats. The 1986 Omnibus Budget Reconciliation Act passed by Congress ordered a $1.5 billion dollar cut in Medicare expenditures by 1989. The Health Care Financing Administration (HCFA) instituted a number of strategies developed by their consultants to accomplish this reduction. Some of the strategies threatened the chief source for funding of medical physics services: the physics Current Procedural Terminology (CPT) codes. Officers of the ACMP visited with congressional leaders and HCFA officials in Washington, DC. These visits were successful in preserving the physics codes and the dollar values assigned thereto; however, the 1990s were to see increasing pressure to end physicians "fee-for-service" billing, which threatened the existence of the physics service codes.

2.4. Highlights of the 1990s

From 1990 through 1998, there was not only continued pressure from the federal government to lower health care costs, but also the rise of health maintenance organizations (HMOs). Mostly publicly owned, these for-profit organizations are driven by return-on-investment concerns. Where HMOs control patient populations, decisions as to the resources necessary for quality patient care rest not on the traditional patient welfare concerns but on return on investment. Because the cost of medical physicists' services constitutes a significant portion of the cost of equipment operation, these costs are closely scrutinized when equipment purchases are evaluated for cost effectiveness. As long as reimbursement for physics procedures is identified with the work performed by the medical physicist, the medical physicist can be justified as a producer of net revenue, rather than a significant item of cost.

3. Funding the medical physicist

Medical physics services are rendered to two consumer groups: 1) directly to the management of a radiological imaging or therapy facility and 2) indirectly through a physician to a patient presenting for diagnosis or treatment. Services rendered to management of a facility are largely standardized, at least on a state-by-state basis, being dictated by safety and regulatory requirements. Billing for these services by privately practicing medical physicists is negotiated in fixed-price contracts or the services may be rendered by salaried medical physicists of a hospital.

In most hospitals associated with medical schools, the medical physicists rendering patient services are salaried, with some receiving augmentation from the physician's patient-care billings. Few of these medical physicists are familiar with how the medical physics services are charged and reimbursed or the implications for budgeting. Medical physicists working in private or community hospitals are more directly involved with the billing procedure, and some have monthly variations in their remuneration when it is based on total billing for physics procedures.

It is important for the medical physicist to be familiar with the details of the institution's billing process. Billing for medical physics and dosimetry services provided for radiation therapy patients is routinely done using a hospital or technical charge referred to as Part A of Medicare charges. Additional details on the CPT codes used for these services have been provided by Richard G. Lane, Ph.D. in the chapter entitled "Medical Physics Staffing Requirements for Radiation Oncology Physics Services." Billing for medical physics services provided for diagnostic imaging and nuclear medicine patients is not routinely done, as explained by Stewart C. Bushong, Ph.D. in the chapter entitled "Medical Physics Staffing for Diagnostic Imaging."

The medical physicist is a unique entity in the hospital setting in a number of ways. Except in Texas and Florida, medical physicists are unlicensed professionals whose educational attainment requirements are equal to or in some cases greater than that of the physician under whose direction he or she works. The medical physicist is uniquely trained to perform machine calibrations and must take full responsibility for the results of this work because error detection cannot be assumed by others. Because there are only about 4000 medical physicists working in clinical areas in the United States, they have little or no political clout, and it is difficult to accomplish legislation on their behalf.

Despite the foregoing, the average salary of the professional clinical medical physicist is roughly equal to that of scientists in commercial and industrial areas and significantly greater than that of a university professor. This situation has not come about naturally but rather through a great deal of effort in structuring physics charges by the leaders in the early days of the profession. Whether or not this trend continues depends on the foresight of today's leaders.

4. Funding in the future

The structuring and subsequent defense of physics charges have spanned the years from 1970 to the present. Recognition of the physics charges provided the fiscal basis for the growth of the medical physics profession. Although the medical physicist has no political clout on the basis of numbers, clout with hospital administrators is gained through recognition of the sizable amount of patient revenues generated by physics activities. It is important that association of these revenues with the medical physicist not be lost, because the physician and the hospital are now targets of stringent "health care cost containment" efforts. Physicist-generated funds must be identified separately to escape strategies designed to reduce physician and hospital costs. It is not the intent of Congress to lower the quality of care patients receive from nonphysicians but rather to cut spending on unnecessary services and fraudulent billing practices.

Of approximately 300 million people in the United States, 38 million are currently Medicare recipients. In an attempt to control expenditures by layering legislation onto legislation each year, Congress has created a situation wherein an incredible amount of paperwork is required to keep the system afloat. To extricate itself from the complexity of overseeing contractors who make payments to providers for millions of procedures on individual patient claims, the HCFA is now putting into place machinery to enable conversion to "managed care" by contracting with HMOs to provide health care to groups of Medicare patients for a fixed dollar amount per patient each year. Several states have begun the process of contracting with HMOs to provide medical services to Medicaid patients on such a capitated basis. The risk is great that the medical physicist's contribution to health care may be obscured in the future. This risk can be managed by taking three very important steps: 1) extending licensure to other states with large populations such as California and New York; 2) identifying the professional clinical medical physicist as a nonphysician health care provider through Medicare legislation; and 3) identifying billing codes for services rendered exclusively by the medical physicist, i.e., continuing medical physics consultation and special medical physics consultation, independent of the physician's codes.

If the profession of medical physics is to continue into the next century as it is known today and the additional quality of care received by the patient through physics services is to continue, medical physicists must address the risks inherent to the changing pattern of health care provision.

Appendix A - The Role of the Health Care Financing Administration

The role of the Health Care Financing Administration (HCFA) is to administer the payment of benefits for medical care as specifically legislated by the United States Senate and House of Representatives. This medical program of government payment for health care was first passed into law in 1965 as an extension of the Social Security Act and is termed the "Medicare Act."

The Medicare payment system was intended to reimburse hospitals for their costs in providing medical care for the aged or financially indigent. Funds are appropriated from the federal budget yearly into Medicare Trust Fund A. The Medicare program is an "entitlement" program; a citizen paying social security taxes is automatically entitled to hospital benefits upon reaching the age of 65. For the financially indigent, a state-administered program called "Medicaid" was established.

The HCFA was created by the Medicare Act to administer distribution of the trust funds. Whereas the enabling legislation is written in very general terms, HCFA is charged with writing specific policies and rules for disbursing funds to providers of health care services. Whereas social security benefit checks are issued directly by the United States Treasury, HCFA contracts with insurance carriers to process claims and issue checks directly to the hospital provider of health care services. Through a system of bids and contracts, an "intermediary" is established for each state.

In a successful effort to stave off nationalized health care, physicians rallied behind extension of Medicare to Part B, reimbursement of physicians for services rendered to patients. The Part B Trust Fund is maintained by assessing each Part B beneficiary a monthly premium, which, while initially set at $3.50, is currently about $45.00. There is also a deductible that must be paid by the individual before benefits start. The Part B Trust Fund is used to contract with carriers to process claims and make payments to physicians and certain other health care providers.

A contract is awarded by HCFA to the successful bidder/carrier from which reimbursement is made for individual patient claims. Unexpended funds remain with the carrier as profit; hence it is in the carrier's best interest to limit reimbursement as closely as possible. Medicare attempts to "standardize" payment across states and individual carriers by periodically issuing Medicare Bulletins defining which services will be reimbursed and which are disallowed. Additionally, the carrier is required to employ the services of a physician to arbitrate disputed claims (such as whether a service is "medically necessary"). Despite these attempts at uniformity, significant differences in reimbursement patterns are found from state to state as a result of exercise of discretion by the individual carriers in payment decisions.

The Medicare chain of authority interdigitates with the federal government budget writing and appropriation process:

The United States Congress:
- passes entitlement legislation by amending the Social Security Act
- passes enabling legislation by amending the Medicare Act
- passes an Omnibus Budget Reconciliation Act (OMBRA) to establish the budget for the following fiscal year, beginning September 1

The OMBRA:
- appropriates funds
- defines what categories of health care providers are eligible to submit claims for reimbursement
- sets limits on total reimbursement in various categories and establishes penalties for violations. The 1997 act established severe punishment such as fines and incarceration for physicians found guilty of violations.

The HCFA:
- writes policies and rules for reimbursement of health care costs
- contracts with *intermediaries* to reimburse hospital providers and *carriers* to reimburse physicians and outpatient centers
- audits payments for violations and fraud
- pursues congressional mandates to lower health care costs

Tables 1 and 2 illustrate the chain of authority.

Table 1. United States Legislative Branch

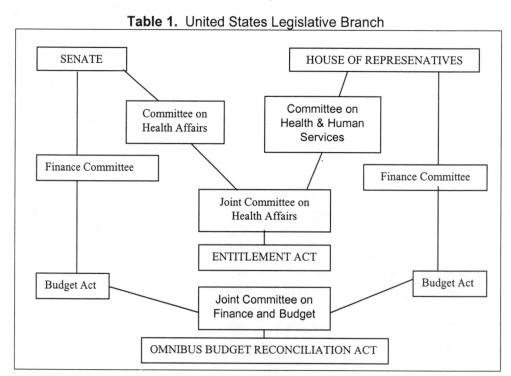

Table 2. United States Administrative Branch

```
┌──────────────────────────────────────────────────────────────────────────┐
│              ┌─────────────────────────────────────────────┐              │
│              │    Department of Health and Human Services    │              │
│              │           Secretary, Donna Shalala            │              │
│              └─────────────────────────────────────────────┘              │
│                                                                            │
│              ┌─────────────────────────────────────────────┐              │
│              │      Health Care Financing Administration     │              │
│              │    Administrator, Nancy-Ann Min DeParle       │              │
│              └─────────────────────────────────────────────┘              │
│                                                                            │
│                    ┌─────────────────────────────┐                        │
│                    │       REGIONAL OFFICE         │                        │
│                    │          Dallas, TX           │                        │
│                    └─────────────────────────────┘                        │
│                                                                            │
│  ┌─────────┐  ┌─────────┐  ┌─────────┐  ┌─────────┐  ┌─────────────┐       │
│  │  Texas  │  │Louisiana│  │ Arkansas│  │ Oklahoma│  │ New Mexico  │       │
│  │ CARRIER │  │ CARRIER │  │ CARRIER │  │ CARRIER │  │   CARRIER   │       │
│  └─────────┘  └─────────┘  └─────────┘  └─────────┘  └─────────────┘       │
└──────────────────────────────────────────────────────────────────────────┘
```

Note: Carriers reimburse insurance claims from Part B Trust funds to freestanding centers, physicians, and other selected nonphysician providers in the state. Hospitals have some choice in the selection of an intermediary who will administer payment of their insurance claims.

Rising public outcry to limit government spending has given rise to passage of annual legislation to limit Medicare spending for health care. In September 1982, the Tax Equity and Fiscal Responsibility Act introduced numerous changes in the historical fee-for-service method of reimbursement. This act was responsible for:

- instituting the prospective payment system for inpatients
- establishing fixed payment amounts for Diagnosis Related Groups in hospitals
- requiring detailed cost reporting by hospitals of expenses incurred in caring for patients
- establishing fixed outpatient reimbursement at prevailing rates
- disallowing many indirect costs and narrowing payments to specific patient services

The December 1986 OMBRA contained provisions that:

- stipulated physician's "usual and customary" charges must fit a vaguely defined classification of "reasonable"
- ordered a 1.5 billion dollar cut in Medicare expenditures by 1989

In order to distribute the cuts in physician reimbursements across the different services, Medicare commissioned a study to establish a "relative value scale" to equate the cost of services performed by family practitioners, internists, pediatricians, surgeons, radiologists, and other medical disciplines. Known as the "Resource Based Relative Value Scale," the final report produced by Abt Associates Inc., Cambridge, MA, utilized information from physician surveys as to the resources required, degree of difficulty, cost of maintaining an office, and other factors to develop an elaborate equation for calculating relative values for all physician services.

Implementation of the study by HCFA resulted in issuance of "allowable" charges to each physician with some disciplines receiving increased reimbursement (family practitioners and internists) and others (such as surgeons and radiologists) receiving drastic cuts. Enforcement of the "allowable" system required standardization of charges, and the American Medical Association was commissioned to publish a "Common Procedural Terminology" for services rendered and procedures performed by hospitals and physicians. This publication is updated yearly, and is known as the "CPT codes." The codes are used in preparing Medicare insurance claims, and have been adopted almost universally by commercial insurance payers as well. A rigid set of criterion are applied to determine if and where a service or procedure fits in the set of CPT codes with graduated "relative value" and thus reimbursement amount.

Although widespread fraud has not been demonstrated, HCFA has expended considerable computer and manpower effort to carefully track payments to providers. In a recent announcement, the Administrator proclaimed that punishment of violators would be the focus of the coming years efforts.

Ann E. Wright, PhD

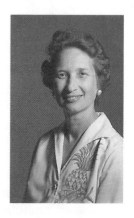

Ann E. Wright received her PhD in Biomedical Sciences (Radiological Physics) in 1970 from The University of Texas Graduate School of Biomedical Sciences, Houston, TX. From 1970 to 1978, Dr. Wright was Chief Physicist and Associate Professor of Radiation Physics at Baylor College of Medicine in Houston. From 1978 to 1992, she was Chief Physicist and Professor of Radiation Oncology at The University of Texas Medical Branch, Galveston, TX, where she is presently Adjunct Professor of Radiation Oncology. Dr. Wright is currently a self-employed medical physics consultant, providing services to hospitals, physicians, regulatory agencies, and industry. Dr. Wright has been a leader in the professional activities of medical physicists. She has served on numerous committees of professional societies, as President of the AAPM, as Chairman of the ACMP, and as Secretary of the American Board of Medical Physics. Dr. Wright was instrumental in helping Texas become the first state to adopt medical physicist licensure. Dr. Wright has received numerous honors for her professional service. She is a Fellow of the AAPM and ACMP and has received the AAPM Southwest Chapter Robert J. Shalek Award and the ACMP Marvin M. D. Williams Professional Achievement Award. Dr. Wright has been very active in communicating medical physics billing information to the HCFA.

Managed Care: What is it?
The Projected Impact of Managed Care on Medical Physics

Geoffrey S. Ibbott, PhD

Department of Radiation Medicine, University of Kentucky Medical Center,
Lexington, KY

Abstract. Managed care is the term used to refer to the organization of hospitals, physicians, and other providers into groups with the goal of enhancing the quality and cost-effectiveness of health care. Managed care is not a new idea. In fact, the United States health care system has been reinvented several times since the 1800s. Modern managed care grew out of early benevolent societies, and programs such as the Kaiser Foundation got their start in the 1930s. This paper reviews the currently available types of insurance coverage, such as traditional third-party fee-for-service payer, preferred provider organizations, health maintenance organizations, Medicare, and Medicaid. Popular terminology and acronyms are defined. Recent trends in health care reimbursement, access, and staffing levels are described. The benefits and liabilities of managed care are discussed with regard to the patient, the health care provider, and the health maintenance organization. How hospitals and private practices are responding is assessed, as well as the impact of managed care on industry. Changes in relationships with health care insurers (payers) are requiring health care providers to modify their staffing patterns, and changes in the medical physics job market are being observed. An assessment of the impact these changes will have on medical physicists is made.

1. Introduction

Medicine has been affected a great deal recently by a phenomenon known as "managed care." Trying to define and understand managed care is not a straightforward task; it is a rapidly evolving process and one whose meaning depends on when and whom you ask. Perhaps one of the best definitions was suggested by Edward Hughes, MD, MPH: "Managed care is the process of the application of standard business practices to the delivery of health care in the traditions of the American free-enterprise system." It is important to remember that managed care is not an isolated cause of the current changes in medicine but the result of changes in society and business. It is equally important to understand that managed care is not a temporary phenomenon to be endured or ignored until it goes away. It is safe to say that managed care is here to stay, although its form will undoubtedly continue to change rapidly. Consequently, medical practitioners of all types, including medical physicists, must understand and adapt to managed care. In this way, we can hope to not only survive managed care but even benefit from it.

Those who have tried forecasting changes in health care have concluded, as Yogi Berra might have put it, "Predictions are very difficult, particularly when they involve the future" (Janower 1973). Trying to anticipate the effects managed care might have on the medical physics practice in the future is similarly difficult. Managed care is a continuously evolving phenomenon, subject to changes in direction driven by industry and modifications and restrictions imposed by legislative authorities in response to consumer reaction.

2. What is managed care?

The term "managed care" describes the organization of hospitals, physicians, and other providers into groups with the goal of enhancing the quality and cost-effectiveness of health care. It is important to recognize that the current incarnation of the managed-care phenomenon is not the first foray down this path in American history. In fact, managed care as we know it today is the latest in a series of periodic structural transitions of the American health care system. The roots of current managed-care programs, including capitation and integration plans, are found in the benevolent societies that were set up in the 1800s (Friedman 1996).

3. Early managed-care experiments

A particularly noteworthy experiment into managed care was the formation of the community cooperative hospital in Elk City, OK. The facility opened in 1931 and was the first capitated physician-hospital organization in the United States. Physicians in the community formed a corporation that built the hospital and sold subscriptions to members of the community. In exchange for their subscriptions, the subscribers were guaranteed all necessary health care at the hospital. The Elk City Community Cooperative Hospital ceased to be a cooperative in 1965 believing that universal coverage had been achieved with the introduction of Medicare and Medicaid.

Another noteworthy managed care venture is the Kaiser Permanente Health Plan. The current Kaiser Permanente Health Plan grew out of a capitated program developed for the Grand Coulee Dam workers in the 1930s. A number of capitated programs for dam workers followed the Grand Coulee project.

Modern managed care is an integrated delivery system that actively manages health services rather than passively financing them (Weiner 1994). Critics of today's managed care often characterize it as "managed cost" or "managed reimbursement," because care is less managed than redirected due to payment restrictions. The cornerstone of managed care is a proactive payment scheme that may range from sharply discounted fees for services to capitation. Discounting fees for services is a direct approach to lowering costs. Capitation, which will be defined later, is a new and different mechanism. One of its attractions is that it motivates physicians to reduce costs. This form of payment represents a fundamental change in the health care business model.

4. The impact of managed care

As of July 1995, 54 million Americans (21% of the population) were enrolled in a health maintenance organization (HMO). It is predicted that by the year 2005, 50% of the American population will be enrolled in some type of managed-care plan. Those who promote managed care believe that the enrollment of half the population will lead to a 20% reduction in health care costs based on 1995 costs. It is estimated that annual increases in health care costs have been reduced by approximately 2% per year as a result of managed-care enrollments. Whether or not these reductions will continue in the future is the subject of much debate (Ginzberg 1997).

5. Managed-care terminology

It may be useful at this point to define some of the terms used in this article.

- HMO: a managed-care organization that provides prepaid, comprehensive coverage for both physician and hospital services. Costs are contained by contracting with the providers who patients are required to use. Large HMOs can demand discounts on drugs and services to further reduce costs.

- Capitation: the payment of a set fee to a health care provider in return for rendering services to a specified group of potential patients.

- Medical-loss ratio: the percentage of health-plan revenue that is spent on payments for medical services. This is an interesting choice of words, because paying for medical services for which the organization exists is considered a loss.

- Preferred-provider organization: a health plan that offers members better benefits if they use providers who have contracted with the plan

- Exclusive provider organization: similar to a preferred-provider organization except that patients receive no reimbursement if they use providers outside the network

- Gatekeeper: a primary-care provider who is responsible for coordinating a patient's medical care. Patients are expected to see the gatekeeper first; the gatekeeper then decides if the services of a specialist are needed.

- Point-of-service plan: a plan to keep costs down by encouraging members to use gatekeepers, limit expensive specialist services, and use providers from the network

6. Examples of managed-care organizations

Presently, two-thirds of employed workers are covered by managed care. Some organizations provide membership in an HMO as a benefit of employment. Many health care organizations have established their own managed-care entities, frequently HMOs, for their employees. Perhaps the most visible contemporary example of the embodiment of managed care in the United States is Columbia HCA Hospital Corporation.

7. Managed-care models

According to Rodwin (1995), managed care appears in one of two forms: the consensus model or the conflict model. In the consensus model, the goals of managed care are mutually reinforcing, and the interests of patients, providers, and payers are compatible. In conflict models, patients, providers, and payers have distinct, sometimes incompatible interests. In general, managed-care organizations have multiple diverging goals, for example, they are concerned with reducing expenditures and use of services, increasing efficiency, eliminating unnecessary treatment, providing better treatment, expanding the range of services, and improving patients' quality of life. Despite the varied manifestations of managed care, there are some shared, essential features (Enzmann 1997).

- Restricted choice of provider: This is the most painful feature for physicians and patients. The purpose of this feature is not better patient care; rather, it is cost control. It is also the feature most likely to change in the future.

- Extensive review of the medical care delivery process by peers and, more importantly, nonpeers: This feature is difficult for physicians to accept because they must agree to the concept that nonphysicians, and possibly patients, are going to measure and judge their performance and quality.

- Negotiable prices; shared risk: This philosophy is in keeping with cost reduction. Physicians now bear financial risks; they once bore only financial security.

- Patient-group model: Rather than serving a select patient clientele, physicians now practice in groups and are responsible for the health care of a defined population. The solo practice of medicine with a selected patient population is a relic of the past.

- The relationship between medical services and the function of insurance companies: The delivery of medical services and the insurance function are tightly linked to managed risk. The closeness of this relationship approaches full integration under the capitation model. These features are likely to undergo modification, but they will continue to define medicine in the forseeable future.

The economic dynamics are well illustrated by AT&T Corporation's switch from a traditional insurance plan to an HMO (Enzmann 1997). The reason was simple. AT&T's health care costs were over $2 billion per year and increasing at more than 10% (Winslow 1996). To reduce this increase in costs, AT&T chose an exclusive contractor, U.S. Health Care, which has the reputation of being a restrictive managed-care company. To help meet their goals, AT&T needed to push its white-collar managers into the HMO. They offered the managers three options: the U.S. Health Care plan, another HMO plan with less desirable features, and a traditional insurance plan. Compared with the HMOs, the traditional insurance program was exorbitantly expensive. The careful packaging of these health care options made the choice so obvious that 85% of the eligible managers signed up with U.S. Health Care.

8. Why managed care now?

Probably the single most important reason for the recent rapid growth in managed care in the United States is the oversupply in the medical marketplace. Excess capacity in the medical care system is the key element enabling purchasers of medical care to force medicine into managed-care arrangements (Ginzberg and Ostow 1997). At the same time, the perceived value of health care is low. Value is judged as the ratio of quality to cost, and consumers, sometimes justifiably, believe that quality has decreased while at the same time costs have escalated. For example, health care spending in the United States increased 6% each year between 1960 and 1990. This has caused health care spending to quadruple from $250 billion in 1980 to $1 trillion in 1995 (Fuchs 1997). Administrative costs have increased also from 24.8% in 1990 to 26% in 1994 (Altman and Shactman 1997). For-profit hospitals spend about 8% more than public hospitals on their administrative costs (Woolhandler and Himmelstein 1997).

It has been estimated that there may be an oversupply of as much as 30% of physicians in the United States in the next 10 years (Ginzberg 1997). Others have estimated that the oversupply of specialty physicians may be as high as 60% by the year 2000 (Weiner 1994). At the same time, others have predicted that the physician surplus will be insignificant in the year 2000 and nonexistent by the year 2020 (Cooper 1995; Friedenberg 1996; Janower and Sunshine 1996). Obviously, there is a great deal of confusion in the physician community; however, a number of other trends are clear (Muroff 1996).

Medicare and Medicaid reimbursement has been declining in recent years, and recent decisions by the Health Care Financing Administration indicate that further reductions, at least in radiology and radiation oncology, are forthcoming (Ginzberg 1997). There have been similar reductions in reimbursement from third-party carriers. Overall, there has been a decrease in the number of procedures for which reimbursement is made and the average level of complexity for which reimbursement is made.

The impact of managed care has been to shift the financial risk from the payer to the provider. Rather than the consumer (the patient) accepting the responsibility for purchasing health services or purchasing insurance for those health services, capitated managed-care programs force the provider to, in effect, become the insurer and accept the financial risk that a large demand for medical services will bring.

There is no question that managed care has reduced the cost of health care. In fact, managed-care plans have become so successful that they have accumulated enormous amounts of liquid assets (in the billions of dollars) and have admitted that they do not know what to do with all the money (Anders 1994). It is unlikely that the public, government, or business will allow them to keep up this profitable pace.

The economics behind this accumulation of revenue are quite simple. The health plan profit margin is determined as total revenue minus administrative costs minus the cost of medical services. The actual payments for medical services vary considerably, as is shown in Table 1 (Enzmann 1997; Smolowe 1996). The managed-care industry uses the term "medical-loss ratio," which was defined earlier, as it has been carried over from the traditional insurance industry in which coverage payments were considered losses. However, continued use of the term gives the impression that revenue is considered profit first and that paying providers for services rendered to health plan members is considered a loss. The medical-loss ratio determines the profit margin. If a health plan has a medical-loss ratio of 80%, it means 80% of revenues go to paying for medical services and 20% goes for marketing, overhead, taxes, and profits (Enzmann 1997). Estimating the typical profit margin may be made as follows.

> Group Health Cooperative of Seattle, WA, a nonprofit organization, has a medical-loss ratio of 91.5%. Other nonprofit HMOs typically have high medical-loss ratios: 89% for Harvard Pilgrim Health Care and 95% for Kaiser Permanente Health Plan. The average for-profit HMO has a medical-loss ratio of 77.4% (Enzmann 1997). Some medical-loss ratios are as low as 60%, and one plan in New Jersey reached 59%. If nonprofit organizations such as Kaiser Permanente can hold their medical-loss ratio to 90% to 95%, administrative costs for these plans can only be in the 5% to 10% range. The administrative costs of Medicare are known to be only 2%. Therefore, health plans incurring loss ratios in the range of 60% to 80% might easily have profit margins of 20% to 30% or even more.

It is expected that the medical-loss ratio for HMOs will increase in the future. As health plans enroll older and sicker patients, spending on care must increase. Growth can no longer be fueled by simply skimming the market for the most favorable customers.

HMOs can limit their medical-loss ratios through capitation. Under this system, a provider is paid a fee on a per-member per-month (PMPM) basis. It is left to the provider to furnish the medical services and split up the monthly lump-sum payments. Splitting the fee among physicians is based on market-determined PMPM rates. Some representative PMPM rates are shown in Table 2 (Enzmann 1997; Scharffe 1995). For some specialties, Medicare, with its older insured population, pays considerably more than commercial HMOs.

Health care consumers, who are better educated and more cognizant than ever before, have begun to make new demands for expanded services and extended hours of service. The competition for provision of services has increased, and this competition comes both from within individual practices and outside those practices.

Another trend that has become apparent is the tendency toward formation of larger physician practice groups.

Table 1. Variation in Average Per-Member Per-Month Payments by New York Health Plans

Health plan	Inpatient hospital care	Physician care
Health Insurance Plan	$60.83	$43.63
Managed Health	$57.78	$30.37
Travelers	$52.92	$83.77
Sanus	$49.67	$64.29
Aetna	$34.77	$52.63
CIGNA	$32.38	$45.53
Choice Care	$31.97	$49.87
Oxford	$31.08	$68.25
MetLife	$29.84	$54.37
U.S. Health Care	$29.05	$41.34
PruCare	$27.78	$50.10
Empire HealthNet	$19.86	$30.61

Table 2. Variations in the Per-Member Per-Month (PMPM) Capitation Rates by Specialty*

	Commercial services average PMPM	Medicare services average PMPM
Anesthesiology	$3.777	$4.647
Cardiology	$1.209	$6.451
Cardiology (invasive)	$0.039	$3.254
General surgery	$1.461	$8.473
Obstetrics and gynecology	$3.662	$2.189
Oncology	$0.869	$3.970
Ophthalmology	$0.684	$5.240
Orthopedics	$1.345	$3.721
Neurology	$0.404	$0.862
Psychiatry/mental health	$2.277	$2.182
Radiology	$2.623	$8.817
Urology	$0.513	$2.066

* The average of 298 HMOs (surveyed in 1995) is compared with Medicare.

9. Trends in radiation oncology

Figure 1 illustrates the change over time in the number of active members of the American Society for Therapeutic Radiology and Oncology (ASTRO). Although the

United States population has increased at a steady but relatively slow rate, it is apparent that the population of radiation oncologists has increased much more rapidly, particularly in recent years (Hussey et al. 1996). The demand for medical services is not strictly a function of the change in total population. The population of the United States is increasing at a rate of approximately 1% per year. However, the average age of the United States population also is increasing, and this aging of the United States population is likely to increase the demand for medical services another 0.5% per year. It has been shown that the availability of newer medical technologies spurs an increase in the demand for those technologies. This trend is presently reflected in an increase in demand for medical services of 4% per year. This is apparent in radiological imaging, where new technologies such as magnetic resonance imaging have driven the increase in demand for services. This phenomenon does not appear to exist in radiation oncology. However, the incidence of cancer also is increasing at approximately 3% to 4% per year. Consequently, with no consideration taken for changes in demand for health care services as a result of managed care, it appears that the demand for imaging and therapy services could be expected to increase approximately 5% to 6% per year.

Active Membership in ASTRO

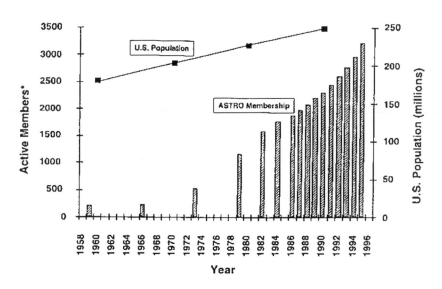

Figure 1. Active membership in ASTRO compared with United States population from 1958 to 1996. Courtesy of ASTRO, Reston, VA.

Another feature of the American health care system has caught the attention of bureaucrats and managed-care providers. The differences in provision of medical services between the United States and other countries is quite startling. Table 3 shows a comparison between the United States, Canada, and other countries in terms of the utilization of radiotherapy and the typical staffing and equipment availability in those countries (Hussey et al. 1996). It is clear that the United States leads much of the rest of the world in terms of the number of patients treated with radiotherapy, the number of radiation oncologists per capita, and the number of megavoltage treatment machines per capita. Interestingly, the number of radiological physicists per capita is approximately equal in the United States and Canada and only slightly less throughout the rest of the world.

Table 3. Comparison of Personnel and Equipment Resources for Radiotherapy in 22 countries* (1991 data)

Number per million population	United States	Canada	Median of 22 countries (including U.S. & Canada)
New cancer patients/yr	~4000 Pts	~4000 Pts	~4000 Pts (range = 1200 - 4600)
Pts treated with radiation therapy/yr	~1800 Pts	~1400 Pts	~1400 Pts (range = 200 – 2400)
No. of radiation oncologists	9.6	6.1	6.75 (range = 0.60 – 23.8)
No. of radiological physicists	3.6	3.6	3.1 (range = 1.1 – 8.5)
Radiation therapists (technologists)	28.4	14.4	14.4 (range = 1.1 – 28.4)
Megavoltage machines	10.3	4.5	3.45 (range = 0.5 – 6.4)
Linear accelerators	8.0	2.5	2.15 (range = 0.2 – 4.6)
Cobalt–60 units	2.3	1.7	1.45 (range = 0.2 – 3.8)

*   Austria, Belgium, Canada, Czechoslovakia, Denmark, France, Germany, Greece, Hungary, Italy, Ireland, Netherlands, Norway, Portugal, Finland, Spain, Sweden, Switzerland, Turkey, United Kingdom, and the United States
Pts, patients

10. Impact on medical physics positions

The rate of growth of the United States medical physics population is illustrated in Figure 2. Over recent years, the number of full members in the American Association of Physicists in Medicine (AAPM) has increased steadily at approximately 5% each year. This rate of increase is largely due to the productivity of medical physics training programs, which, in 1994, turned out 180 graduates. However, it is expected that the annual productivity of these programs will reduce to roughly 100 graduates per year in 1998 (Paliwal 1996).

The demand for medical physics positions is very likely dependent on a number of parameters that are outside our control.

• The number of radiology and radiation oncology procedures performed annually

• The number of radiologist and radiation oncologist positions

- The introduction of health care legislation mandating (or potentially prohibiting) medical physics services (e.g., the Mammography Quality Standards Act, thought to have increased the demand for medical physics services considerably)

- Changes in reimbursement patterns, as well as Current Procedural Terminology (CPT) code relative values, which may change the availability of medical physics positions

- The degree to which medical physicists are perceived to provide a "value-added" service to health care

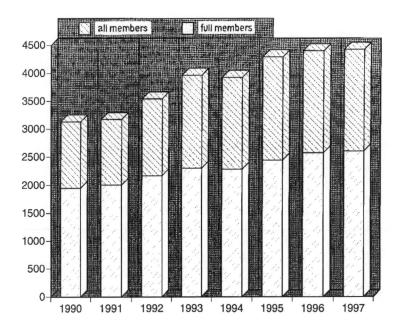

Figure 2. Number of full AAPM memberships between 1990 and 1997

The available data are not very encouraging. In 1995, for the first time, medical physics salaries, corrected for inflation, decreased slightly over the previous years, as illustrated in Figure 3. These data were taken from the annual AAPM professional survey and were published in mid-1996 (American Association of Physicists in Medicine 1995). Although not graphed in Figure 3, the average reported salary in 1996, without correction for inflation, was $90,600. This is a 2.5% increase over 1995, which may again have been erased by inflation.

11. Projections for the supply and demand of medical physicists

The preceding data have been used to make a crude estimate of changes in the supply and demand for medical physics services over the next few years. The graph in Figure 4 compares the projections for growth in the supply of medical physicists with the projected demand for medical physics positions. Two curves are shown for both supply and demand, representing the maximum and minimum credible rates of increase of each. The first curve indicates the supply of medical physicists if the present rate of growth of the profession is allowed to continue. As indicated earlier, the present rate of growth is 5% per year; so the 1995 full membership of the AAPM of approximately 2,400 physicists would increase to over 4,000 physicists in the year 2006. However, if the supply of medical physicists is restricted to 2.5% growth per year after 1997, then a lower curve results. Two curves indicate the demand for medical physics positions based on an optimistic growth rate of 4% per year (assuming no impact of managed care on the growth and demand for health services) and a pessimistic growth rate of 2% per year. It has been estimated previously that managed care is likely to reduce the growth in demand for medical services by 2% per year. All four curves intersect in the year 1995. This reference point was deliberately chosen as possibly representing a recent state of ideal balance between the supply and demand for medical physicists. From this figure, it appears that a controlled growth of the medical physics profession might coincide ideally with a growth and demand for health care that falls between the most optimistic and most pessimistic projections.

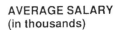

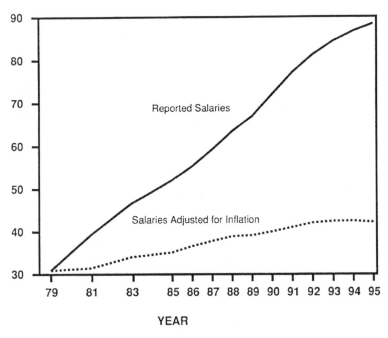

Figure 3. Average principle salary of AAPM members from 1979 to 1995. Solid line, reported salary; dashed line, salaries adjusted for inflation using Consumer Price Index – All Urban Consumers (CPI-U). Courtesy of AAPM, College Park, MD.

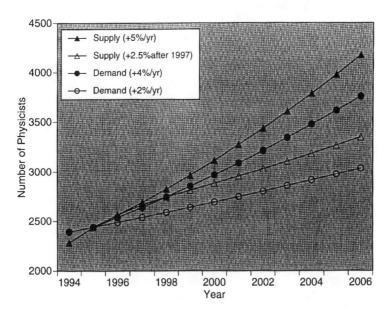

Figure 4. Projections of supply and demand for medical physicists from 1994 to 2006.

12. Strategies for medical physicists

What strategies are available for medical physicists in the face of possibly reduced demand for our services and increased competition from colleagues? The way I see it, we have two alternatives: we can resist or we can adapt. If we choose to resist, we had better prepare ourselves for a career in a nonmedical field. If we choose to adapt, there are several issues we should probably consider carefully.

- Physicists most likely will have to make sacrifices similar to those being made by other health care providers. Some physicians are accepting lower salaries or lower salary increases; in other cases, they are accepting reduced working hours.

- Medical physicists should consider finding new and innovative ways to accomplish the work required at a lower cost. This may involve the use of computers to generate reports, the substitution of a new piece of equipment with greater capabilities for a more antiquated piece of equipment, or even redesigning work procedures for a more streamlined approach.

- The correct utilization of appropriately trained staff can be used to reduce the resources required for a given task.

- Our training programs must monitor the market for medical physicists.

151

13. The image of the medical physicist

A key technique for surviving under managed care centers around the image of the medical physicist in the clinic. It is well understood that many medical physicists have difficulty looking at how they might be perceived by other health care professionals. Unfortunately, in this arena of managed care, medical physicists who are not seen as critical to patient care run the risk of being eliminated by administrators with sharp pencils. A survey performed by Task Group 7 of the Professional Information and Clinical Relations Committee of the AAPM uncovered some surprising and rather disturbing facts about the behavior of many medical physicists (American Association of Physicists in Medicine 1995). Shown in Figure 5 is a chart indicating the distribution of time of a number of medical physicists who were surveyed by the task group (Dawson 1995). Shown on one axis is a short list of common responsibilities of clinical medical physicists. These include direct patient care, interacting with the physician, interacting with the dosimetrist, interacting with the therapist, and working in one's own office. On the other horizontal axis are breakdowns of the percent of time spent in each activity, and on the vertical axis are the number of physicists who reported each activity and a corresponding time interval. Of concern is the appearance that medical physicists tend to spend the greatest amount of time in their own offices and the smallest amount of time interacting with the therapist or with the physician. Slightly greater amounts of time are shown spent interacting with the dosimetrist or in direct patient care. However, it is my opinion that physicists who spend the majority of their time working privately in their own offices run the risk of being overlooked when decisions are made regarding the allocation of resources.

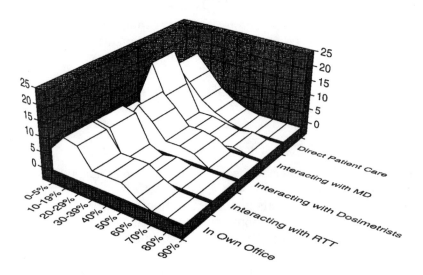

Figure 5. Results of a survey by Task Group 7 of the AAPM Professional Information and Clinical Relations Committee: Number of respondents versus time they spend for the activities indicated.

In addition, medical physicists must pay attention to several key issues as the oppressive characteristics of managed care roll across the health care scene.

- Medical physicists must maintain professional standards in the face of reduced or altered demand for our services.

- We must be careful to maintain our relationships with the physician community, because medical physicist positions are so dependent on the demand physicians make for our services.

- Physicists must be seen as realistic and interested in responding to the needs of the clinic. It does us no good whatsoever if we appear aloof or uninterested in the interests of the physicians and therapists.

Physicists must clearly demonstrate the value added by their presence in the institution. Our survival depends in no small part on our ability to convince administrators and physicians that the quality of health care services provided by our institutions would be seriously and negatively impacted by our removal or replacement. We must be highly visible in the clinic, must be actively involved in the day-to-day activities, and must convey an impression of interest and concern in the future of the institution.

References

Altman SH and Shactman D (1997) Should we worry about hospital's high administrative costs? *New England Journal of Medicine* **336** 798-799

American Association of Physicists in Medicine (1996) "President's Column: Addressing the impact of change." *American Association of Physicists in Medicine Newsletter* July-Aug, **21**(4),1-2

— (1995) "Professional information survey report, Calendar year 1995" Woodbury, NY:AIP

Anders G (1994) HMOs pile up billions in cash, try to decide what to do with it. *The Wall Street Journal* Dec 21,A1

Cooper RA (1995) Perspectives on the physician workforce to the year 2000. *Journal of the American Medical Association* **274**,1534-1543

Dawson J (1996) Cost justification survey results, *American Association of Physicists in Medicine Newsletter* May-June, **21**(3),9

Enzmann DR (1997) Surviving in Health Care. St. Louis, MO:Mosby-Year Book Inc.

Friedenberg RM (1996) Future physician requirements: Generalists and specialists—Shortage or surplus. *Radiology* **200**,45A-47A.

Friedman A (1996) Capitation, integration, and managed care: Lessons from early experiments. *Journal of the American Medical Association* **274**,957-962

Fuchs VR (1997) Managed care and merger mania. *Journal of the American Medical Association* **277**,920-921

Ginzberg E and Ostow M (1997) Sounding board: Managed care—A look back and a look ahead. *New England Journal of Medicine* **336**,1018-1020

Ginzberg E (1997) Managed care and the competitive marker in health care: What they can and cannot do. *Journal of the American Medical Association* **277**,1812-1813

Hussey DH, Horton JL, Mendenhall NP, Munzenrider JE, Rose CM, and Sunshine J (1996) Manpower needs for radiation oncology: A preliminary report of the ASTRO Human Resources Committee. *ASTRO Newsletter* **133**,1-14

Janower ML (1973) Too many radiologists? *Radiology* **108**,219-221

Janower ML and Sunshine JH (1996) Too many radiologists? Update. *Radiology* **200**,545-549

Michaels JW (1988) Thoughts on the business of life (Editorial). *Forbes* Sept 19,224

Muroff LR (1996) Health care reform and radiology. *Radiology* **199**,39A-43A

Paliwal B (1996) Addressing the impact of change. *American Association of Physicists in Medicine Newsletter* July-Aug, **21**(4),1-2

Rodwin MA (1995) Conflicts in managed care. *New England Journal of Medicine* **332**,604-607

Scharffer DL (1995) What is imaging's role in the managed care world? *Diagnostic Imaging* Dec, **34**

Smolowe JA (1996) Health merger. *Time* **147**,77-79

Weiner J (1994) Forecasting the effects of health care reform on U.S. physician workforce requirements: Evidence from HMO staffing patterns. *Journal of the American Medical Association* **272**,222-230

Winslow R (1996) Switch to HMO care can be turbulent, as AT&T case shows. *The Wall Street Journal* May 9,A1

Woolhandler S and Himmelstein DU (1997) Cost of care and administration at for profit and other hospitals in the United States. *New England Journal of Medicine* **336**,769-777

Geoffrey S. Ibbott, PhD

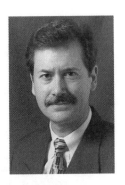

Geoffrey S. Ibbott received his MS degree in Medical Physics from the University of Colorado Health Sciences Center in 1981, and he received his PhD in Radiation Biology from Colorado State University in 1993. Dr. Ibbott has worked as a medical physicist in the Department of Radiology at the University of Colorado Health Sciences Center (1974 to 1990) and as a radiological physicist in the Department of Therapeutic Radiology at the Yale-New Haven Hospital (1990-1993). In 1994, Dr. Ibbott took his current position as Associate Professor and Director of Physics in the Department of Radiation Medicine at the University of Kentucky Medical Center. Dr. Ibbott is well known for his contributions to educational and professional activities. He was director of the University of Colorado Graduate Training Program in Medical Physics from 1981 to1986, and he has been a member of the faculty of the Medical Physics Training Program at the University of Kentucky since 1994. Dr. Ibbott has been very active in the professional aspects of medical physics. He has served as chairman of the AAPM Professional Council (1993 to 1997), chairman of the Subcommittee on Accreditation of Regional Calibration Laboratories (1996 to present), and president or president elect for three different chapters. In 1999, he became President of the AAPM. He has served on the Board of Directors and on multiple committees and councils and was honored as Fellow in 1996. He has also served on numerous committees of the American College of Radiology and was Counselor at Large in 1996, 1997, and 1998. He has been active in a number of societies and served as a liaison for the Trilateral Committee to the Joint Commission on Accreditation of Health Care Organizations from 1994 to 1997. As part of his ongoing interest and leadership in professional issues, Dr. Ibbott presented a talk on managed care at the 1996 American College of Medical Physicists Professional Symposium, clearly showing his understanding of this issue.

The Profession of Medical Physics and Malpractice Issues

Robert J. Shalek, PhD, JD

Department of Radiation Physics, The University of Texas M. D. Anderson Cancer Center, Houston, TX

Abstract. The professional lives of physicians who use radiation in medicine and of physicists who provide radiation sources in useful form have been tightly intertwined in their 100-year history and continue to be so. In the last 50 years, a debilitating competition between physicians well trained in the medical use of radiation and other more generally trained physicians who use radiation has been largely resolved in favor of the specialists. Physicists and engineers have played an important role in that competition by the development of equipment and techniques that require use by medical specialists. As radiation oncologists, diagnostic radiologists, and nuclear medicine physicians have prospered, so have medical physicists. In recent years, the number of lawsuits arising from medical diagnosis and treatment have increased. A unified approach by physicians and medical physicists is recommended to reduce the probability of malpractice lawsuits and to effectively handle lawsuits that do occur. I recommend that medical physicists assume responsibility for the quality of imaging machines and the correct fulfillment of radiation prescriptions in therapy.

1. Introduction

From the discovery of x-rays and radioactivity by physicists in the 1890s, the professional lives of physicians who use ionizing radiation and the professional lives of medical physicists who provide the radiation sources and detectors in a clinically useful form have been intertwined; thus, these professionals have been mutually dependent. A characteristic of medical physics that may distinguish it from biomedical engineering is the continuing and regular need for participation of medical physicists in the practice of therapeutic radiology, diagnostic radiology, and nuclear medicine. At the 1997 annual meeting of the American Association of Physicists in Medicine (AAPM), over 98% of the presentations appeared to be related to these radiation medical specialties. In the first part of this paper, I will review some well-known historical facts concerning radiation professionals and the relationship between medical physicists and physicians practicing radiological medicine. In the last part of the paper, I will consider medical malpractice and responses of the physician-physicist team.

2. A short history of radiation professionals in the United States

From 1900 to beyond 1950, physicians in the United States who called themselves diagnostic radiologists, therapeutic radiologists, or both competed with other established medical specialists in the medical use of radiation. Radiation was promoted by equipment suppliers and others as a tool that could be used by most medical specialists. Just as any licensed physician could do surgery, any licensed physician (and in the early days even unlicensed staff) could use radiation in medicine. Physicians in general practice, internal medicine, and various types of surgery very often had diagnostic x-ray sets in their offices and performed their own diagnostic radiology tests; surgeons, gynecologists, dermatologists, and urologists performed radiotherapy principally with radium sources but sometimes with 200 kVp x-rays.

From the early 1930s onward, radiologists laid the groundwork for recognition of radiology as a viable medical specialty when the American Board of Radiology (ABR) instituted certification guidelines for radiologists and other subspecialties in 1934 (Knight 1996). By 1937, of 68 "class A" medical schools in the United States, 40 had chaired radiology departments, and 27 had radiology functions in departments of surgery, pathology, or anatomy. The question of whether radiation oncology and diagnostic radiology should be separate medical specialties was raised in the late 1930s and was carried into the 1970s before an affirmative decision was made. By 1975, training in general radiology (diagnostic and therapeutic) was no longer available (Cox 1996). In 1938, there were 39 radiation oncologists in the United States (Cox 1996). In 1958, the Club of Radiotherapists was formally established with 54 members; later, the name was changed to the American Society for Therapeutic Radiology and Oncology (ASTRO). By 1963, there were 111 full-time radiation oncologists, and by 1983, there were 1600 full-time radiation oncologists (Cox 1996). In 1997, ASTRO had 3157 active members plus about 1600 associate, corresponding, and junior members for a total membership of about 4800.

The increase in the number of medical physicists over time is similar to the increase in radiation oncologists. In 1936, a registry was compiled listing 45 qualified radiation physicists in the United States and Canada (Feldman 1996). Physicists had begun participating in the ABR examination of physicians around 1935. In 1949, an ABR examination and diplomate status in radiological physics was first offered. Between 1958 and 1960, there were 133 charter members of the newly formed AAPM. By 1997, the AAPM had a total membership of 4500 members. In 1982, the American College of Medical Physics was formed, and by 1997, the organization had approximately 450 members. This organization sponsored the American Board of Medical Physics, which began examining medical physicists in 1988. In 1995, 69% of the work done by medical physicists was related to radiation oncology, and 21% was related to diagnostic radiology, magnetic resonance imaging, and nuclear medicine (Tolbert 1997).

3. Mutual dependence

In any place where medical care is given, physicians are the primary caregivers and have legal responsibility to patients for the quality of that care. Medical physicists support radiation oncologists, diagnostic radiologists, and nuclear medicine physicians by providing physics services, research, and training. Likewise, other professionals, such as medical dosimetrists, radiation therapists, and x-ray technologists, similarly provide essential services and are dependent on the physician.

In radiotherapy, a long chain of events is involved in the delivery of radiation from the proper use of calibrated measuring instruments to determining the time or number of monitor units employed in treatment. In most radiotherapy installations, the medical physicist is the only person who can trace and verify the accuracy of all the steps in the chain. Thus, the day-to-day accuracy of the fulfillment of radiation prescriptions depends on the medical physicist, whether or not the physicist is given that explicit responsibility.

The events of World War II (1939 to 1945) stimulated scientific and technical innovations such as self-sustaining nuclear fission, microwave generation for radar, and the digital computer. From just after the war to the present, these seminal inventions have yielded artificial radionuclides, cobalt irradiators, linear accelerators, and many applications of digital computers. The betatron and van de Graaff accelerators have scientific roots preceding the war but came to practical medical use about the same time as the other inventions mentioned. A few medical physicists participated in bringing the wartime inventions into being, and since 1945, many medical physicists have participated in creating medical applications for those and later inventions. Probably almost all medical physicists working in therapeutic radiology have participated in introducing these innovations into regular medical practice in a way that is consistent with previous practices. Likewise, some medical physicists have participated in the development of new imaging systems, and many have participated in placing the innovations into regular use. The cost and skill required in the application of modern imaging technology has enhanced the role of the diagnostic radiologist. Thus, the technical efforts of medical physicists have contributed to the success of radiation oncology and imaging specialties and in recent times have helped physicians in these specialties to outpace other physicians using radiation because of the increased skill and capital investment required. In turn, the radiological medical specialties have returned recognition and success to medical physics. The past 50 years like the first 50 years have been a time of achievement but also have been a time of professional maturing for the radiological subspecialties. Diagnostic radiology, radiation oncology, and nuclear medicine have won respect and a secure position within the professional medical community. Medical physics has achieved similar status within the radiological community.

4. Medical environment

Managed care has brought about increased economic pressures for those in medicine. In private health care, administrators have gained ascendancy because of their ability to attract patients to their institution by making agreements with insurers and others as the medical authority of physicians in some places has declined. Likewise, in some publicly administered health care systems where nonmedical administrators have authority, physicians sometimes find that they are not included in planning, and thus, their ability to fulfill their responsibilities to patients is reduced. But in both the private and public setting, a malpractice event weighs heavily on the physician. In Texas, until 1997, health maintenance organizations (HMO) could not be sued in malpractice cases because they were not practicing medicine and their physicians were contractors, not employees. By Texas statute (the first such state law in the United States), HMOs can now be sued, but the HMOs will contest the statute in the courts. A complication is the existence of the federal Employee Retirement Income Security Act (ERISA), which affects employer-sponsored health plans. ERISA has been ruled in federal court to preempt state law and allow recovery only of the cost of the health benefit denied and not personal damages resulting from the lack of medical treatment (McGinley 1998). Time will need to pass before this situation is clarified in the courts or by legislation. I advise physicians, medical physicists, and other professionals in radiation medicine to remember their history and to make decisions that best benefit patients and that preserve their responsibility toward patients while effecting economies. Business-like relationships that recognize the responsibilities and contributions of each person on the radiological team are crucial to establishing and presenting a unified position to management.

5. Physicist responsibility

AAPM Report No. 33 (American Association of Physicists in Medicine 1991) and Report No. 42 (American Association of Physicists in Medicine 1994a), both of which relate to diagnostic radiology, clearly recommend that the medical physicist be responsible for the quality of images. However, the AAPM position regarding radiation oncology is not as clear. AAPM Report No. 38 (American Association of Physicists in Medicine 1993) states that "the physicist is responsible for the physical accuracy of the dose delivered." AAPM Report No. 40 (American Association of Physicists in Medicine 1994b) recommends that "the overall responsibility for a machine quality assurance program be assigned to one individual: the radiation oncology physicist." This recommendation sounds similar to that recommended in Report No. 38, but it carries a lesser responsibility. Taken literally, Report No. 40 implies that following an approved checklist for machine quality assurance is sufficient on the part of the medical physicist. If the list appears as a governmental regulation, then the force of law would undergird the checklist. I do not want to minimize the value of checklists, but I believe that a checklist for a machine quality assurance program does not ensure the physical accuracy of the dose delivered in every instance. Human error, misinterpretation of dose prescriptions, and new or altered techniques might introduce errors that a machine quality assurance program would not reveal. On a Radiological Physics Center site visit, I once found that a radiation oncologist and a medical physicist had disagreed on what was being done in a certain complex treatment. To resolve the question, I watched as a radiotherapist treated a patient using the technique in question and noted that what was done in the treatment was not what either the physician or the physicist had suggested.

Employers are liable for the actions of their employees in the course of their work. Problems arise when plaintiff's lawyers or defendant's insurance companies in a malpractice suit attempt to identify what went wrong in a radiotherapy treatment regimen. The lawyers and insurance companies are interested in spreading blame, particularly if the participants who planned and executed the treatment are employed by different entities, such as a physicians group, a hospital, or a medical physics consultation group. Cases in which there is faulty communication between the persons implementing treatment or in which more than one error occurred are likely to involve blame-fixing to determine who pays. I have noticed that regardless of the outcome of a malpractice suit, the radiological team often breaks up with people leaving the organization. I speculate that this result occurs because of ill will arising from efforts to fix responsibilities after a defining event rather than before. In this instance, I recommend that each person involved in fulfilling the dose prescription understand and acknowledge their responsibilities and that one person have responsibility for the integrity of the complete chain of events and, indeed, the delivery of the correct dose to each patient, thus following the guidelines of AAPM Report No. 38.

The medical physicist is usually the person most capable of assuming overall responsibility. The medical physicist may have direct supervisory responsibility for medical dosimetrists, radiotherapists, machine engineers, and others. If that is not possible because of institutional history, seniority, or other reasons, giving the medical physicist an overall auditing role may work. A medical physicist who has the firm support of management in an auditing capacity may have sufficient authority to ensure the correct fulfillment of radiation-dose prescriptions. Under this system, the medical physicist would always bear responsibility for an incorrectly filled radiation prescription except, perhaps, in the case of a catastrophic machine failure. An analogous responsibility for imaging physicists is to ensure that an imaging system meets or exceeds a national standard of care. For example, the Mammography Quality Standards Act (U.S. House of Representatives 1992) in federal regulations defines the training requirements of various personnel and quality assurance equipment tests required for performance of mammograms. Medical physicists should follow pertinent regulations but should realize that more than just following regulations may be required to define the standard of care by a court in a malpractice case, particularly if there are circumstances beyond those contemplated by the regulations (Shalek and Gooden 1996).

6. Negligence

A physician acquires responsibility to the patient through the formation of a physician-patient relationship. As hospitals became more involved in patient care, starting about 30 years ago, hospitals acquired responsibility to patients through a legal theory called "direct corporate liability." Medical physicists usually acquire responsibility to patients as employees or agents of a physician or hospital (or radiation center). The employer is "vicariously liable," that is, fully responsible in a legal action based upon a medical physicist's negligence. However, be aware that an employer can seek "indemnification," that is payback, from an employee for damages paid to a plaintiff resulting from negligence of the employee, providing the employer was not also negligent.

By far the most likely legal theory to be applied against medical professionals is negligence. A patient-plaintiff must prove four elements of negligence by a preponderance of the evidence in order to prevail in a malpractice lawsuit:

- That the duty of a medical professional is defined by a standard of care
- That the duty was breached
- That the breach of duty caused injury
- That the injury resulted in damage to the patient

People who present themselves as radiation professionals should have the education, knowledge, and experience to understand and perform according to a national standard of care. That standard of care is defined through the general literature, governmental regulations, reports by professional organizations, usual practice elsewhere, and common sense. Further discussion of negligence related to medicine is available (Shalek and Gooden 1996).

7. Policies to forestall a suit or improve a defendant's position

All persons involved should be encouraged and are legally obligated to challenge the procedures that they and others perform that could harm a patient. An extended discussion of the legal basis for both of these policies is presented by Shalek and Gooden (1996). Thus, contradictory policies appear to be recommended here, namely that each person have clear responsibilities; that the medical physicist have concurrent, overall responsibility for imaging quality and fulfillment of radiation prescription in therapy; and that each person have responsibility to expose errors and inconsistencies in their work and the work of others. Good leadership can make such a system work by considering errors "objective events" that can be dealt with rather than as "personal failures." Personalizing errors has lead to cover-ups and concealments that in turn have lead to harm to patients under treatment or to confusion in the radiation oncologist's association of dose prescription and clinical result, leading to less-than-optimum radiation prescriptions for future patients.

More particularly, policies put in place for quality assurance, if administered thoughtfully, can go far to forestall events that could lead to a malpractice suit. Such policies should include redundant checking at critical points in the chain of events of radiotherapy. For example, passive checking of the time or monitor units in radiation delivery by external beam answers a recurrent question: Do the treatment records reflect what was actually done? Having an independent in-house staff member check treatment plans for errors is important. Having an independent outside person or agency check machine calibrations is usually acceptable evidence of correct machine operation without bringing forth extensive calibration protocols. In diagnostic radiology, the ability for a medical physicist or a responsible person to demonstrate that on any day an imaging system, more probably than not, was operated to a national standard may prove important in future controversies. Diagnostic radiologists are the most sued physicians on a legal theory sometimes called "lost chance due to delayed diagnosis." Mammography screening is often involved. I am unaware of a legal suit against a medical physicist for lost chance due to a poorly operating imaging machine, but such a theory is likely to come. A discussion of quality assurance principles and references is provided elsewhere (Shalek and Gooden 1996). The time and effort spent to ensure quality assurance is costly, often repetitive, and not greatly interesting, but the extended concentration required of a defendant in a malpractice suit is far greater and much more unpleasant.

Soon after the discovery of an event that could result in a legal suit, it is important that: 1) the responsible designated person (usually the department head) be notified promptly, 2) patient records be protected, and 3) the result of the event on the patient or patients under treatment be fully understood before machine changes and corrections are instituted (Shalek and Gooden 1996).

Decisions regarding subsequent handling of a situation that may become the basis of a lawsuit usually do not fall to the medical physicist, but a physicist may be able to provide useful advice. The medical physicist's input might include one or more of the following.

Questions:

- Is it possible to compensate in the remaining treatment for an underdose or overdose?

- How does the radiation dose delivered compare with prescribed doses at other institutions?

Suggested Actions:

- Notify administration; urge involvement of their legal counsel.

- Notify the insurance company in the manner and within the time they require.

- Notify the radiation control agency if and when required.

- Notify referring physicians and the patient. Inform the patient of the possible health-related implications.

- Recommend no charge to patient for ameliorative medical treatment. Such treatment or offers of compromise cannot be used as evidence to prove liability for injury according to Federal Rules of Evidence 408 and 409 (Shalek and Gooden 1996).

- Be aware that subsequent remedial measures to improve a machine or a procedure cannot be used as evidence to prove negligence in a prior event according to Federal Rule of Evidence 407 (Shalek and Gooden 1996).

- The legal counsel of a hospital may recommend reporting the results of investigations to a hospital committee in order to control the timing of media reports.

8. Additional professional comments

In small to medium-sized radiation treatment or imaging groups, the organization is usually not greatly important, because each person will be recognized for their contribution and the responsibility they bear. In larger institutions where in addition to the clinical responsibilities the physicists also may report to graduate schools and granting agencies, organizational clarity is likely to be important.

At a minimum, medical physicists usually perform the following professional functions.

- Create technical innovations or at least integrate commercial innovations into existing systems

- Correctly fulfill radiation therapy dose prescriptions and ensure some level of responsibility for the performance quality of imaging machines (I believe medical physicists should seek full responsibility for these functions.)

- Train employees, physician residents, and medical physics students

It is important for physicists to be aware of the following.

- Radiation oncologists, diagnostic radiologists, and nuclear medicine physicians must be satisfied with the medical physics services they employ in their practice.

- Medical physicists should be legally informed in order to protect their employer and themselves as far as possible from legal missteps.

- Some physicians and some medical physicists are sometimes arrogant. The physician is most likely to err in trying to cast the medical physicist in a technician role, and the medical physicist is most likely to err in believing that his or her higher learning confers an exalted status apart from their actual role. When the posturing stops, the ingenuity, the reliability, and the responsibility borne by an individual find recognition in respect and usually competitive salary.

In imaging, medical physicists make a contribution that will almost certainly continue and likely increase. As long as radiotherapy continues to be prescribed, the role of the medical physicist will continue and will likely increase. There have been many predictions concerning the solution of the cancer problem. In 1913, an institution that specialized in cancer treatment was said to have built a temporary building because they expected a solution to cancer to be forthcoming. Now, however, with technologies that enable the rapid detection of genetic mutations in individuals, a broader understanding of the causes of cancer may be at hand, but utilizing that information in newer, more focused therapies may be a long and difficult road. I do not feel qualified to put these possibilities in perspective; however, I recommend a chapter by Herman Suit that discusses this topic (Suit 1996).

References

American Association of Physicists in Medicine (1991) "Staffing levels and responsibilities of physicists in diagnostic radiology," AAPM Diagnostic X-ray Imaging Committee Task Group 5 Report No. 33. Woodbury, NY:AIP

— (1993) "Statement on the role of a physicist in radiation oncology," AAPM Report No. 38. Woodbury, NY:AIP

— (1994a) "The role of the clinical medical physicist in diagnostic radiology," AAPM Report No. 42. Woodbury, NY:AIP

— (1994b) "Comprehensive QA for radiation oncology," AAPM Report No. 40 *Medical Physics* **21**,581-618

Cox JD (1996) Clinical practice. RA Galiardi, JF Wilson, and N Knight, eds. A History of the Radiological Sciences: Radiation Oncology. Reston, VA:Radiation Centennial Inc., p 21-42

Feldman A (1996) 1915-1934. RA Gagliardi and PR Almond, eds. A History of the Radiological Sciences: Radiation Physics. Reston, VA:Radiation Centennial Inc., p 51-83

Knight N (1996) Training and education. RA Gagliardi, JF Wilson, and N Knight, eds. A History of the Radiological Sciences: Radiation Physics. Reston, VA:Radiation Centennial Inc., p 1-20

McGinley L (1998) Broad battle to end HMO's limited liability for treatment-coverage denials gains steam. *The Wall Street Journal* Jan 12, A22

Shalek RJ and Gooden DS (1996) Medical Physicists and Malpractice. Madison, WI:Medical Physics Publishing

Suit HD (1996) The future of radiation oncology. RA Gagliardi, JF Wilson, and N Knight, eds. A History of the Radiological Sciences: Radiation Oncology. Reston, VA:Radiation Centennial Inc., p 293-312

Tolbert D (1997) Medical physics practice trends from salary survey data. *American Association of Physicists in Medicine Newsletter* Jan-Feb, **22**(1),11-12

US House of Representatives (1992) "Mammography Quality Standards Act of 1992," H.R.6182, Public Law 102-539 (106 Stat. 35478), October 27, 1992; Interim Rule (58 FR 67558) December 21, 1993; Amendment (59 FR 49808), September 21, 1994. Washington DC: US House of Representatives.

Robert J. Shalek, PhD, JD

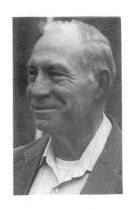

Robert J. Shalek received a master's degree in Physics and a PhD in Biophysics from the Rice Institute (now Rice University) in Houston, TX in 1953. While working on a doctoral degree, he held the position of Assistant in Physics at The University of Texas M. D. Anderson Hospital and Tumor Institute (now The University of Texas M. D. Anderson Cancer Center) in Houston. From 1953 to 1954, he was a postdoctoral research fellow under Professor W. V. Mayneord at the University of London Royal Cancer Hospital (now the Royal Marsden Hospital) in Sutton, Surrey, England. Dr. Shalek accepted a faculty position at M. D. Anderson in 1954, where he attained the rank of Professor of Biophysics in 1961. He served as Chairman of the Department of Physics from 1961 until his retirement in 1984. Dr. Shalek has an impressive research and publication record in radiation chemistry, brachytherapy dosimetry, and quality assurance related to radiotherapy. He was active in the formation of The University of Texas Graduate School of Biomedical Sciences at Houston and the degree and nondegree programs in Biophysics and Medical Physics. He supervised five doctoral candidates, three master's degree candidates, and several postdoctoral and nondegree students. Management at M. D. Anderson strongly encouraged serving the community at large in various aspects of medicine. In medical physics, Dr. Shalek was the founder of such opportunities which included: giving short courses in medical physics with open registration, which began over 40 years ago and continues today; providing technical support to medical physicists in isolated areas of Texas; and establishing the Radiological Physics Center, which was instrumental in implementing national radiotherapy physics standards. For his contributions to medical physics and radiotherapy, Dr. Shalek is a Fellow of the AAPM and has received the highest award offered by three professional societies: the AAPM William D. Coolidge Award, the American College of Medical Physics Marvin M. D. Williams Award, and the ASTRO Gold Medal. Late in his career, Dr. Shalek studied law at night school, received a law degree in 1983, and was admitted to the Texas Bar. Since retirement, he has remained Professor Emeritus at M. D. Anderson and has served as consultant, expert witness, and lecturer in legal issues related to medical physics.

Technical References

Technical Information and Reports for Medical Physicists

Peter R. Almond, PhD

Department of Radiation Physics, The University of Texas M. D. Anderson Cancer Center, Houston, TX

Abstract. There is a large amount of technical information available to the medical physicist, ranging from state and federal regulations to journals, newsletters, reports, meeting proceedings, and textbooks. State and federal regulations help define the required standard of care, and medical physicists need to be familiar with all pertinent regulations that apply to their work. Additional helpful information can be obtained from the organizations that provide input to the regulators, i.e., the National Council on Radiation Protection and Measurement and the Conference of Radiation Control Program Directors. Scientific societies such as the American Association of Physicists in Medicine publish scientific journals, reports, and meeting proceedings, which contain useful technical information, often relating to new or innovative techniques. The publications of the various professional colleges also contain helpful material. Standard medical physics textbooks can also be used as useful resources. In addition, various government and private organizations issue newsletters and information sheets on technical subjects. Much of this information is on the Internet, but caution must be used when accessing unrefereed material. By careful planning, the medical physicist can keep up-to-date on all the latest technical developments.

1. Introduction: How much information is there?

This paper will discuss where professional medical physicists can find the technical information they need to perform their jobs. Most of the information will relate to radiation oncology and medical health physics, but the basic principles can be applied to diagnostic radiology, imaging, nuclear medicine, and other areas of clinical physics.

The primary sources discussed here are printed information. Although the Internet is a popular and much-used information resource, care must be taken when using this information, because much of it will not have been reviewed or verified with the exception of official government reports or electronic journals.

2. Regulations: The standard of care

In *Medical Physicists and Malpractice,* Shalek and Gooden (1996) state:

> "If a medical physicist complies with a regulation, that regulation may fully define the standard of care expected from the activity addressed, but a high standard could be defined and justified in a trial for negligence."

What this means is that the regulations help define the standard of care. In general, because the standard of care will go beyond the regulations, the physicist must be aware of and comply with all pertinent regulations to provide a minimum level of care. The regulations cover a wide range of subjects including basic radiation protection requirements, radioactive materials, x-ray-producing machines, and reporting of misadministration.

The regulations are established by two sources: the federal government and the state government. States that have agreed to base their regulations for by-product material on federal regulations are called "agreement states" and will have a state department for radiation matters. The term "by-product material" for medical purposes refers to radioactive material obtained from reactor fission material or materials activated in a reactor. Kentucky and Texas are agreement states. In Kentucky, the Radiation Control Branch of the Cabinet for Human Resources issues two documents: Radioactive Material Regulations and Radiation Producing Machines. In Texas, the Bureau of Radiation Control in the Texas Department of Health issues a single document, Texas Regulations for Control of Radiation, which covers all areas. More than half the states are now agreement states.

Those states that do not wish to regulate the use of by-product material themselves are called "non-agreement states" and are regulated directly by the Nuclear Regulatory Commission (NRC) of the federal government. The NRC issues its regulations in the "Code of Federal Regulations" (CFR), primarily in two parts: 10 CFR Part 20, "Standards for protection against radiation," and 10 CFR Part 35 "Medical use of by-product material." Copies of these documents can be obtained directly from the NRC or downloaded from the NRC World Wide Web site.

Part 35 includes the Quality Management Program, the Misadministration Rule, and the requirements for a Radiation Safety Committee and Radiation Safety Officer at medical institutions. Medical institutions using radioactive materials must be licensed either by the state or by the NRC.

Another federal agency that issues regulations concerning radiation is the Food and Drug Administration (FDA). In particular, the FDA has been involved with regulations concerning mammography; 10 CFR Part 900 is the Mammography Quality Standards Act.

Medical physicists should be familiar with all pertinent federal and state rules and regulations. It is good practice when submitting a contract for medical physics services to use the appropriate state and federal regulations as a basis for the proposed work.

3. Keeping one jump ahead: With whom do regulators consult?

Although regulators, both state and federal, draw on many sources, several sources are used consistently: the National Council on Radiation Protection and

Measurements (NCRP), the Conference of Radiation Control Program Directors (CRCPD), advisory committees, and scientific and professional organizations.

The NCRP is a nonprofit corporation chartered by Congress in 1964 to collect, analyze, develop, and disseminate, in the public interest, information about protection and measurement of radiation; to cooperate with all organizations to develop basic concepts; and to consult with international and governmental bodies concerned with these matters. The NCRP issues reports (Report No. 125, "Deposition, retention, and dosimetry of inhaled radioactive substances," was published in February 1997), commentaries, proceedings of meetings, and lecture series. The NCRP tends to follow very closely the recommendation of the International Commission on Radiological Protection which, also issues reports.

The effect of the NCRP reports on regulations can be seen from the following example. In NCRP Report No. 39, "Basic radiation protection criteria," issued in 1971, the annual dose limit for the public was set at 0.5 rem (5 mSv). This dose limit was used in NCRP Report No. 49, "Structural shielding design and evaluation for medical use of x-rays and gamma rays of energies Up to 10 MeV," and Report No. 51, "Radiation protection design guidelines for 0.1-100 MeV particle accelerator facilities," to set the design criterion for noncontrolled areas (i.e., public areas) as 10 mrem (0.1 mSv) per week. This number was incorporated into NRC and state regulations as the design goal for shielding of all medical radiation facilities. However, in Report No. 91, "Recommendations on limits for exposure to ionizing radiation," issued in 1987, the NCRP revised its recommendations for the annual dose limit to the public to 100 mrem (1 mSv). Subsequently, the NRC and then the states changed the design criterion for the noncontrolled areas to 2 mrem (0.02 mSv) per week. This change has had a significant impact on the thickness of shielding barriers for medical radiation installations.

The NCRP also can be requested to provide information for regulatory purposes. In a petition to the NRC, the America College of Nuclear Medicine asked for a rule change for the release of patients administered radioactive material. The NRC turned to the NCRP for advice and recommendations on the problem of exposure of family members and members of the public due to contact with patients receiving radionuclide therapy. In 1995, the NCRP published Commentary No. 11, "Dose limits for individuals who receive exposure from radionuclide therapy patients." The NRC then changed their regulations to reflect the recommendations from the NCRP but not before the proposed rule change was published for public comment in the Federal Register and discussed by the NRC's Advisory Committee on the Medical Uses of Isotopes. The states then followed the NRC and changed their regulations.

The states, in addition to the NRC, generate proposed regulations through the CRCPD. The CRCPD publishes "Suggested state regulations for the control of radiation" out of its Frankfort, KY office. This is a dynamic document that is changed as frequently and as quickly as possible as new revised parts become available and is endorsed by the NRC, Environmental Protection Agency, and the FDA. This document is much broader than the NRC regulations, which by law are limited to by-product material. "Suggested state regulations for control of radiation" deals with all aspects of ionizing and nonionizing radiation, including x-ray-producing equipment and medical linear accelerators. The "Suggested state regulations for the control of radiation" can be and are often used by the states as models for their regulations.

Information concerning the NRC, FDA, NCRP, and CRCPD can be found at the appropriate sites on the World Wide Web (www.nrc.gov, www.fda.gov, www.rsna.org/about/orgs/ncrp.html, and www.crcpd.org, respectively).

4. How to keep up-to-date: Why review the literature?

In the context of this paper, "literature" refers to journal articles, reports, proceedings, and similar types of information sources. A list of some of the journals that target medical physicists or that publish articles relevant to medical physics (in English) are listed in Table 1. These journals are generally published by scientific and medical societies. These organizations also publish newsletters and proceedings of topical symposia, summer schools, etc. Many of the equipment manufacturers publish their own newsletters and proceedings of users' meetings, which may prove helpful when initiating new clinical procedures.

Groups like the NCRP and the International Commission on Radiation Units and Measurements (ICRU) publish useful information in their reports, several of which are produced each year. The following examples show the usefulness of these resources.

- Initiating multileaf collimator use: This practice includes dosimetric considerations such as output calculations and effects on dose distribution. In recent years, many excellent articles have appeared in scientific journals such as *Medical Physics* and *Physics in Medicine and Biology*.

- Starting total-skin electron therapy: In addition to the many other excellent articles in the literature, the American Association of Physicists in Medicine (AAPM) published Report No. 23 on total-skin electron therapy as well as covering the topic in some of the summer school proceedings.

- Planning intra-ocular eye implants: The proceedings of the AAPM 1994 summer school session on brachytherapy includes a comprehensive paper on this subject.

- Knowing the correct definition of treatment volumes for conformal therapy: This can be found in ICRU Report No. 50.

Table 1. Journals and Sponsoring Organizations

Journal	Sponsoring Organization
Medical Physics	American Association of Physicists in Medicine
Medical Dosimetry	American Association of Medical Dosimetrists
Radiotherapy and Oncology	European Society of Therapeutic Radiation and Oncology
The British Journal of Radiology	British Institute of Radiology
Physics in Medicine and Biology	Institute of Physics and Engineering in Medicine
International Journal of Radiation Oncology, Biology, Physics	American Society of Therapeutic Radiology and Oncology
Radiation Research	Radiation Research Society
Health Physics	Health Physics Society
Radiology	Radiological Society of North America
Journal of Nuclear Medicine	Society of Nuclear Medicine
Endocurietherapy/Hyperthermia Oncology	American Brachytherapy Society

5. Back to basics: Should textbooks be discarded?

The textbooks that the physicist studied during training should be kept along with any additional books that might prove helpful. Table 2 lists the topics of some of these textbooks. Over the years, these textbooks can become useful references, especially for procedures, calculations, and concepts that are not carried out routinely. For example, the chapters on discrete radioisotope sources by Loevinger, Japha, and Brownell and internally administered radioisotopes by Loevinger, Holt, and Hine in the textbook entitled *Radiation Dosimetry* (Hine and Brownell 1958) are very helpful in determining the beta-dosimetry for P-32 solutions.

Although *The Atomic Nucleus* by Evans (1955) is not a medical physics textbook, it contains many of the basic physics concepts and calculations that form the foundation of clinical physics. As an example, this book contains the derivation of the build-up factor for a point gamma ray source in an infinite isotropic medium, which is needed for calculating dose distributions around implanted brachytherapy sources.

Table 2. Textbooks That Serve as Useful References for Medical Physicists

Textbook	Author	Publisher
The Physics of Radiation Therapy	Khan	Williams & Wilkins
The Basic Physics of Radiation Therapy	Selman	Thomas
The Physics of Radiology	Johns and Cunningham	Thomas
The Physical Foundation of Radiology	Glasser, Quimby, Taylor, Weatherwax, and Morgan	Hoeber-Harper
Radiation Dosimetry	Hine and Brownell, (eds.)	Academic Press
Radiation Dosimetry, Volumes I, II, and III	Attix, Roesch, and Tochilin (eds.)	Academic Press
The Atomic Nucleus	Evans	McGraw-Hill Book Publishers
Medical Radiation Physics	Hendee	Year Book Medical Publishers
Radiation Therapy Physics	Hendee	Year Book Medical Publishers

6. Leftovers: Was anything left out?

There is a large amount of additional information available, much of which is free or accessible via the Internet. Table 3 lists some of the organizations that routinely publish reports, newsletters, handbooks, and information on the World Wide Web that may be useful to the practicing medical physicist. This list is only representative, and there are many other such publications that might also be useful.

Special mention should be made, however, of the supplements published by the British Institute of Radiology (BIR) on central-axis depth-dose data. First published in 1953 as Supplement 5 of the *British Journal of Radiology*, the information has been revised and updated several times (Supplement 10, 1961; Supplement 11, 1972; and Supplement 17, 1983). The last revision was published in 1996 as the *British Journal of Radiology* Supplement 25, "Central axis depth dose data for use in radiotherapy: 1996." The supplement was prepared by a joint working party of the BIR and the Institute of Physics and Engineering in Medicine and Biology and was published by the BIR. Although this report has depth-dose data for all conceivable therapy beams (eight sections covering x-rays from a half value layer of 0.01 Al to 50 MV, electrons, neutrons, and protons), it is much more. Each section has an excellent introduction covering the characteristics of the radiation in question, and there are six appendices on more general subjects such as the equivalent field method and normalized peak scatter factors. The supplement ends with a useful glossary of terms. These supplements have been the mainstay of radiation oncology departments for years, and the latest edition will prove as useful as its predecessors.

Table 3. Organizations Sponsoring Newsletters, Bulletins, Reports, E-mail Announcements, and Other Important Information Resources

U.S. Nuclear Regulatory Commission, *e.g., Office of Nuclear Material Safety and Safeguards Licensee Newsletter*
Food and Drug Administration, *e.g., Mammography Matters*
International Commission on Radiation Units and Measurements, *e.g., ICRU News*
International Atomic Energy Agency
International Organization for Standardization
International Electrotechnical Commission
National Academy of Sciences - National Research Council, Committee on the Biological Effects of Ionizing Radiation
National Institute of Standards and Technology

7. Discussion: Can it all be managed?

It is clear that there is a large amount of data, technical reports, and information available to the medical physicist. In fact, there is so much information, that it may seem impossible to manage it all. Listed below are several suggestions for helping the physicist keep up-to-date on all the latest developments.

- Obtain a copy of the appropriate state and NRC regulations, and get on their mailing lists for updates. NRC regulations can be found on the Internet. Large institutions or groups should consider purchasing the "Suggested state regulations for control of radiation" from the CRCPD and any subsequent updates.

- Get on the government's mailing list for free bulletins such as "Mammography matters and radiological health bulletins" from the FDA's Center for Devices and Radiological Health; "Nuclear material safety and safeguards licensee newsletter" from the NRC; and the National Voluntary Laboratory Accreditation Program's "News from the national institute for standards and technology."

- Join one of the related physics societies, either the AAPM or the Health Physics Society. Both memberships include a journal and newsletter subscription.

- Join an appropriate clinical society, depending on your main area of work and interest, such as the American Society For Therapeutic Radiology and Oncology, the Radiological Society of North America, or the Society of Nuclear Medicine. In addition, there are other societies that are associated with each of the subspecialties of the three main clinical areas. All of these societies provide journals, newsletters, or both to members.

- Join one of the appropriate colleges: the American College of Radiology, the American College of Medical Physics, or the American College of Nuclear Medicine, each of which publishes bulletins, newsletters, or both.

- Review the publications of the NCRP, the ICRU, the International Commission on Radiological Protection, and the International Atomic Energy Agency. Some of these publications can be useful reference material for day-to-day activities and should be purchased for your personal use.

- Establish a personal library of your textbooks, journals, newsletters, proceedings, and reports.

- Plan to attend at least one national or local meeting a year to keep up with the latest developments.

It may not be possible to do all of the above, but it is important to keep up with the appropriate regulations and developments in you particular area of work and expertise. In order to do this efficiently, it is very important to get feedback on what works and what does not work. Regular meetings with other physicists and chat groups on the Internet will help facilitate this type of interaction.

References

Evans, RD (1955) The Atomic Nucleus. New York, NY:McGraw-Hill Book Company

Hine GJ and Brownell GL (1958) Radiation Dosimetry. New York, NY:Acamdeic Press Inc.

Shalek RJ and Gooden DS (1996) Medical Physicists and Malpractice. Madison, WI:Medical Physics Publishing

Peter R. Almond, PhD

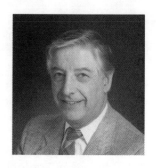

Peter R. Almond received his PhD in Physics from Rice University, Houston, TX in 1965. During his graduate studies, he was the Rice University Fellow in Physics at The University of Texas M. D. Anderson Hospital and Tumor Institute (now The University of Texas M. D. Anderson Cancer Center) in Houston, TX. After a 2-year postdoctoral appointment, Dr. Almond accepted a faculty position in the Department of Physics at M. D. Anderson Hospital and Tumor Institute, where he remained until 1985, serving as Professor of Biophysics and Chief of the Radiation Physics Section from 1972 to 1985. From 1985 to 1998, he served as Professor and Vice Chairman of Research in the Department of Radiation Oncology at the University of Louisville James Graham Brown Cancer Center, Louisville, KY. As an academician, Dr. Almond has published approximately 100 articles with major contributions in electron dosimetry, TLD, ion chamber dosimetry, neutron dosimetry, and brachytherapy. He has taught numerous continuing-education and graduate-education courses, having supervised over 15 master's degree and doctoral candidates. His professional contributions are too numerous to list but are substantiated by his having received two of the highest awards for medical physicists: the AAPM William D. Coolidge Award and the American College of Medical Physics (ACMP) Marvin M.D. Williams Award. Dr. Almond is also a Fellow of the AAPM and ACMP. Dr. Almond is in high demand to serve on committees setting international and national guidelines, having participated on over 20 task groups and scientific committees of the AAPM, NCRP, International Council on Radiology and Protection, and Nuclear Regulatory Commission. At the present time, Dr. Almond serves as Editor-in-Chief of the *Journal of Applied Clinical Medical Physics* and is a Research Professor in the Department of Radiation Physics at M. D. Anderson Cancer Center.

Index

Index

Index

Index